PRAISE FOR
Making Love Again

"...readable, informative and persuasive...glossary, bibliography, resources list and index make this book professionally complete...solidly recommended for public libraries."

The Library Journal

"A remarkable story for both patients and physicians...Virginia and Keith Laken describe what so many must feel when facing the same challenges. Their frank descriptions...have allowed us all to gain insight and how one can indeed face, cope with, and overcome the fears associated with this condition."

David Barrett, M.D.
Chief Executive Officer, Lahey Clinic, Boston, Massachusetts

"*Making Love Again* is an eloquent book that adds to a small but important force in literature about sex in the real world...Virginia and Keith Laken have courageously offered their story so that others may learn what a 'real' couple has done to keep intimacy alive, despite the realities of sexual dysfunction. May reading about their healing help speed your own."

Bob Burns
Producer/Director, The Truth About Impotence, *NOVA 1998*

"In *Making Love Again*, Virginia and Keith describe in intimate detail their struggle with impotence. It is their struggle, even though it's Keith's impotence. Together they recount the various treatments, the anxious moments and the false hopes, the good sex and the bad, the cures that weren't. And they report the corresponding rise and fall of their relationship—all with such unreserved honesty that the book is a genuine page-turner."

Psychology Today

"A ground-breaking book that is a must read for health care providers or anyone dealing with sexual dysfunction, prostate cancer, or lack of sexual intimacy. Should be in all hospital, medical, public and personal libraries."

Chris Kraft, Ph.D.
Johns Hopkins Center for Marital and Sexual Health, Baltimore, Maryland

"This necessary book will help patients and their lovers face problems, identify solutions that work for them and transcend despair. It also will help their physicians understand their patients' experience, be alert to their needs and be quicker to provide professional guidance."

James A. Talcott, M.D., S.M.
Director, Center for Outcomes Research
Massachusetts General Hospital Cancer Center, Boston, Massachusetts

making
LOVE
AGAIN

Hope for

Couples

Facing

Loss of

Sexual

Intimacy

making
LOVE
AGAIN

Virginia and Keith Laken

For permissions and reprint information, contact: vklaken@hopeforcouples.com

Printed in the U.S.A.
First printing, February 2002
Second Printing, April 2002
Third Printing, September 2017

Editor: Maria Bishop
Second Edition Editor: Michelle Urbick
Cover Design: Michelle Urbick

Disclaimer
This book is intended for the general reading public and not as a substitute for qualified medical care. The authors, editors, and publisher are not responsible for errors or omissions, or for any consequences from application of the information in this book, and make no warranty, expressed or implied, with respect to the contents of the publication.

Publisher's Cataloging in Publication

Laken, Virginia
    Making love again : hope for couples facing loss of sexual intimacy /
    Virginia and Keith Laken. — 2nd ed.
    p. cm.
    Includes bibliographical references and index.
    ISBN-13: 978-1543272185
    ISBN-10: 1543272185
    1. Laken, Keith—Health. 2. Impotence—Popular works. 3. Sex—Popular
works. 4. Prostate—Cancer—Patients—Biography. 7. Prostate—Cancer—
Patients—Family relationships. 8. Prostate—Cancer—Patients—Sexual
behavior. I. Laken, Keith. II. Title
RC889.L35 2002   362.1 '96692'0092
                                                    QB101-201456

To my father, Fred Langbehn,
who also faced this condition due to
heart medication side effects.

—Virginia Laken

TABLE OF CONTENTS

OPENING REMARKS

Making Love Again is an eloquent book that adds to a small but important force in literature about sex in the real world.

Together, male and female sexual dysfunction affect as many as half of all individuals between the ages of 40 and 70. I know this because, in 1997, I was hired to produce "The Truth About Impotence" for NOVA, the PBS science series.

At that time, I knew nothing about the issue. Worse, what I thought I knew turned out to be wrong. My ignorance was typical. I knew how stomach acid digested food, blood carried nutrients to cells and neurons passed electrical signals to cause one to feel and think. But how did the penis get hard? I didn't have a clue. I didn't know it was a blood-filled inflatable. I thought it was just a rather odd muscle.

And maybe it doesn't matter much if any of us knows how our genitals work....until they don't.

We would all like to just have a pill to make impotence better, but it doesn't really work that way. Sex is a delicate dance involving complex emotions, psychology and physiology. To heal oneself, one needs to understand that dance. One needs to talk and listen and learn from people who have been through it before.

Within these pages, Virginia and Keith Laken have courageously offered their story so that others may learn what a "real" couple has done to keep intimacy alive, despite the realities of sexual dysfunction.

May reading about their healing help speed your own.

—Bob Burns
Producer/Director *The Truth About Impotence*, NOVA 1998

FOREWARD

In this book is a remarkable story for both patients and physicians: one couple's journey through the roller-coaster ride of dealing with sexual dysfunction as a consequence of prostate-cancer treatment. Within these pages, Virginia and Keith Laken describe what so many must feel when facing the same challenges.

For me, as a urologist, Virginia's recollections point out the role of the physician in understanding a patient's feelings.

From the very beginning of my career in medicine, I, like all physicians, have treated many different patients with many types of personalities. And while people respond to news about their health with varying degrees of emotion and awareness, the fact remains that the bond between health-care practitioner and patient is extremely important in helping the patient deal with the reality of a diagnosis.

When diagnosing erectile dysfunction, explanations must be clear, but compassionate and caring as well. Both patient and physician must accept the fact that some information may not be understood or even heard during the shock of initial coping. Honesty, repetition and caring are paramount.

Physicians must never lose sight of the responsibility they have in dealing with a patient's *emotional* struggle—not just the physical challenges of disease management.

Virginia and Keith, through their frank descriptions of the reality of erectile dysfunction, have allowed us all to gain insight into how one can indeed face, cope with and overcome the fears associated with this condition.

We all will benefit from their sharing this wonderful story.

—David M. Barrett, M.D.
Chief Executive Officer
Lahey Clinic
Burlington, Massachusetts

INTRODUCTION

Although this book is written by my wife, Virginia, it has always been important to Gin and me that this book accurately reflect the story of how the *two* of us learned to deal with—and overcome—impotence.

And how could we think otherwise? Impotence, by its very nature, affects both partners in a relationship, so, logically, any story about it should give equal time to both the male and female voices.

But writing isn't something I'm very good at.

So when we had to decide who would actually put the story on paper, we always knew it would be Gin who would do the actual writing.

This doesn't mean, however, that I sat back while Gin told my story "as she saw it".

I was an active, involved participant in this book, reading and rereading the text as it evolved daily. I frequently critiqued Gin's interpretation, and added and deleted details freely. I included my opinions and corrected her perceptions when I needed to.

Gin and I have spent literally hundreds of hours talking about scenes, dialogue and, most importantly, the journal entries that offer our most personal reflections.

The time and energy we have invested in *Making Love Again*, however, has been worth every second. Not only have we been able to produce a book of which we are both proud, but we've also been able to analyze our own story from a more objective, distanced point of view. Consequently, we feel we better understand our emotional responses to impotence, and we also better appreciate the happiness and joy we currently share in our sexual relationship.

Our goal was always to write a book that focused not so much on the *cause* of impotence but on its *effects*. I would be remiss, though, if I did not at this point acknowledge the reality of my "trigger" for becoming impotent.

Prostate cancer is a deadly disease, and should never be underestimated in its ability to kill. While I feel I'm cured of my disease, I never want to come across as minimizing that threat. I have only the deepest respect and empathy for the thousands of cancer victims who have never had the chance, like I did, to get beyond fighting the disease. I know I'm one lucky guy—and I often find myself embarrassed and humbled by the fact that I've survived while so many others have not.

But I *did* survive, and the question became: Now what do I do with my life?

My hope is that, in part, this book gives back to the prostate-cancer community—and to anyone suffering from impotence. I want others to realize that there *is* hope after becoming sexually dysfunctional.

Life can still be rewarding.

And you can still have great sex!

—Keith Laken

CHAPTER ONE

"That Surgery Can Make A Guy Impotent!"

"Are you *listening* to me? That surgery can make a guy impotent! There's *no way* I'd risk letting that happen to me!"

Keith paced around the kitchen table where I stood watching him. My stomach was churning, and my fingers curled inward so tightly the nails were cutting my palms.

"How can you *say* that?" I demanded, my voice becoming shrill. "How could you even think of risking your *life* for the sake of having sex?!"

We had reenacted this same argument so many times over the past two years. Keith had had two inconclusive biopsies for prostate cancer so far. And while the diagnosis was still unconfirmed, our discussions over the possibility of surgery—and its accompanying risk of impotence—had become recurrent, ambushing us as we attempted to go about our daily lives. Standing in our sunlit kitchen on an ordinary Saturday morning, the conversation seemed almost ludicrous. But it was very real.

"You have such a tough time getting this."

Keith yanked a chair out from under the table and jammed his square-set body into it. "Having sex is what makes a man a man. If a guy can't perform, he might as well hang it up."

"You can't *really* believe that?" I asked. Keith was always so logical, and this departure from reason annoyed me. "Life is not about getting a hard-on! It's about *being* together. Sharing our *lives* with one another."

I moved into the chair nearest Keith, and tentatively touched his arm. "If you have cancer and you don't get rid of it, hon, you're going to die long before you should."

Tears began to fill my eyes for the millionth time.

"Then what would happen?" I asked forlornly. "I'd be left alone. A widow. And *why*? Because *you* want to have *sex!*"

Keith gave me a hard stare, his blue eyes piercing.

"Gin. Listen. To. Me." he said, punctuating each word with increasing precision. "I keep telling you. This is not just about sex. It's about *life*. What kind of *life* would I have if I couldn't make love to you anymore? If I thought people didn't respect me? What kind of *life* would that be?"

Keith's eyes were searching mine, looking for empathy. I tried my best to be consoling.

"Hon, I know sex is important. I *understand* that. But sex isn't *everything*. As long as we have each other, it'll be all right. It's not important to me that we have *sex*," I reassured him, "only that I have *you*."

Instead of offering solace, my words seemed to sting. Keith's face reddened, and he slammed his palms down on the table.

"*That's* nice to hear!" he said sarcastically. "Well *you* might not care about having sex anymore, Gin, but *I* do!"

Gathering steam with each word, he continued, "And if my choice is to live longer and be half a man, or to live a shorter life with all my capabilities, you'd better believe I'd rather live a shorter, more fulfilling life!"

In the silence that followed, we avoided each other's eyes, struggling with emotions we obviously couldn't make the other understand.

When had we turned into people who argued like this?

As this thought crossed my mind, Keith spoke with quiet finality.

"Just get it out of your mind that I would ever have that surgery."

We had been shocked, in January of 1993, when the doctors had first suggested a biopsy. Keith had gone to see Dr. Robert Phyliky, our family doctor at the Mayo Clinic, for nothing more than a yearly check-up.

He was only 47 years old at the time—way too young for prostate cancer. But the blood work had indicated otherwise. Keith's prostate-specific antigen (PSA) level was elevated, and the doctors were suspicious.

When the first biopsy came back negative, we had wanted to believe we were safe. But the experience had been so disturbing we couldn't shake it. Especially Keith. Ever the pragmatist, he had wanted to be prepared just in case, and understand all his options. So he'd started doing some research on prostate cancer and treatment choices.

As he'd assembled information and downloaded reports from the Internet, Keith shared his findings with me. The data was confusing—even, at times, conflicting. The primary treatment options at the time were radiation, surgery or "watchful waiting". And, from the beginning, the two of us had looked at these options from different perspectives. I thought any potential cancer should be totally removed from Keith's body, and, thus, I only had considered surgery. Uncharacteristically, Keith was more cautious. Given the possible consequences of surgery, he stated often that if he *were* to be diagnosed with prostate cancer, he might not consider *any* treatment.

Keith's mindset frightened me. I dug in my heels and continued to push for surgery. And that was when our arguments first began.

It was unusual for Keith and me to have bitter fights. After twenty-seven years of marriage, we had reconciled most of what I thought were our major differences. We still had disagreements, of course, but they were usually over petty things. And while we *did* often debate with each other, this was something we did for pleasure—an exercise in stretching our minds. Our debates were frequently intense, but seldom hostile.

Until the biopsies, I had thought we were at a good point in our marriage. We had moved around a great deal when the children were small, including living in Iran for two years in the 1970s. And while we had both enjoyed this adventurous side of our lives, for the last eight years we'd been happy to settle comfortably in rural Minnesota.

Our home is in a picturesque valley overlooking the Mississippi River, and bald eagles and other wildlife share the property with us. It had felt good to put down roots here, and we were enjoying the relaxed pace of living outside a small town.

Our children, who were teenagers when we first moved to Minnesota, were now grown and living on either coast. With Beth and Steven no longer at home, Keith and I had been savoring the luxury of time alone together. We loved to take long, rambling walks or curl up to watch a good movie. And we were finally beginning to plan a few of those long-discussed "adventure trips."

Yes, life was going smoothly. I had my own business as a part-time communications consultant, which provided me the freedom to visit the children and stay involved in our community. Keith's job as vice president/general manager of the electronics division of his company seemed to offer the perfect challenge: Developing new products and mentoring people were what he did best.

Our marriage was strong and supportive, our health good.

Never did we think that cancer would enter our lives and cause us to start arguing so vehemently.

"If a guy's impotent, he's *powerless!*" Keith railed.

The swiftness with which our conversations changed was amazing. Just minutes before, we had been enjoying a quiet walk in the woods, commenting on the fall colors and laughing over the antics of Kikan, our fox terrier. Now, somehow, we were fighting again. And whenever we discussed cancer or impotence, we lost our sense of humor, digressing quickly into touchy sarcasm that made it impossible to maintain a civil discussion.

"Keith, who could ever think of you as powerless?" I countered sharply.

Stopping in mid-stride, Keith dropped my hand and turned toward me. His face was flushed again, and his brow furrowed.

"If I became impotent and anyone at work ever knew," he said, almost threateningly, "they'd lose their confidence in me. They'd think of me as a useless eunuch!"

I had heard Keith express this concern many times, and I knew it was a real issue for him. But I just didn't get it. Wasn't he the leader of the largest division in his company? The visionary who turned the electronic sector around? More than four hundred people depended on his leadership to keep the plant operating at a profit. How could he ever think his sexual performance would affect people's perception of him?

This made no sense to me.

Ignoring his comments, I tried a different angle.

"Hon, if you have cancer, the important thing is to get cured."

"No, Gin! It's *not* just about curing cancer," Keith shot back, running a hand through his ash-blond hair. "It's about being human. If I couldn't enjoy sex, I'd feel like a freak of nature!"

In this argument, like so many others, we came to no resolution. Instead, I headed back to the house, my shoulders hunched against the wind, supremely tired of this issue that continued to divide us.

Laptop Notes, October 18, 1994

Gin suggested I start keeping a journal, like she does. She thinks maybe it will help me keep track of where I'm at with this whole prostate cancer thing. I'm sure she's hoping it might help me change my mind about surgery if it comes to that.

I don't think that's going to happen.

But I'm on the machine a lot anyway, so I might as well try this.

Journal Entry, October 28, 1994

I don't understand why Keith is being so unreasonable. He's totally convinced he'd become impotent if he had to have this surgery, and no one can make him think otherwise. It's unlike him to be so stubborn...and selfish.

All he seems to be thinking about is his sex life. What about his LIFE?

I know if it were me facing a surgery that might save my life, he'd insist I have it. But somehow he thinks it's different for him.

Arguing over this same issue is exhausting. It's been so unproductive and hurtful.

It's also scary. Keith's life could be at stake.

Laptop Notes, November 2, 1994

Another fight. Gin can be so frustrating.

What kind of a marriage would we have if we couldn't have sex? She's being naïve. Always the Pollyanna.

Steven says if this does turn out to be cancer, the docs he's started working with at Johns Hopkins suggest the operation, too. Easy for them to say. It's not their sex life.

In January 1995, when it was time for Keith's third prostate screening, we were both tired. We had been living in a kind of purgatory, enduring torturous waiting between yearly appointments, and always wondering if this time the cancer would be confirmed. The stress and uncertainty had taken a toll on us, and we talked about making this our last appointment ever.

"I don't want to go through this anymore," Keith insisted as we waited for the head of the urology department, Dr. David Barrett, to come into the examination room. "It's too nerve-racking."

"You know I agree with you, hon. If there's no change this time, even *I'll* say we should stop." I gave Keith a wan smile.

He didn't smile back. Behind his glasses, his eyes looked weary.

"If that guy so much *even hints* at any more tests, I'm gonna lose it, Gin."

Keith picked up a magazine from the rack, while I returned to my paperback. We were seated side by side on the hard, built-in bench connected to the doctor's desk. I was trying my best to appear calm, despite the constant flip-flop in my stomach.

I looked around the examination room. It was standard Mayo Clinic: well equipped for efficiency. We sat in front of a black examining table, which was draped with a white sheet and surrounded by high-tech equipment. The sterility of the environment made it hard to concentrate on the novel I was reading—or to think about anything other than the impending meeting. But I tried my best to focus on a page, and reread the same sentence for the fourth time.

When David Barrett entered the room, I stared at him. I always forgot how handsome he was. With his trim physique and dark hair just beginning to gray, he cut a very distinguished figure. I guessed he was around our age.

When I had first met him, after Dr. Phyliky's referral, I'd thought Dr. Barrett a bit brusque. Like so many surgeons, everything about him had seemed so clinical. By now, however, my opinion had changed; I saw his concern for Keith, and the interest he had in the well-being of his patients. I was even beginning to like him.

Dr. Barrett greeted us, and perfunctorily introduced the two young residents who followed closely behind him. As always, he was quick to get down to business. He asked if he could palpate Keith's prostate before giving us the results of the blood work. Keith grimaced, but agreed. I left the room.

When the brief examination was complete, Dr. Barrett called me back in. He made a few notes in Keith's chart, then looked at us.

The results, he said, were alarming.

Not only had Keith's PSA level risen once more, but Dr. Barrett could now feel a nodule on Keith's prostate. Sure enough, he suggested the dreaded third biopsy.

Keith refused.

Emphatically.

"I'm *not* going to have another biopsy!" he exploded at the white-coated figures. "I feel like a victim here! Like I'm prey to you guys! You're hunters, looking for cancer—and you're determined to find it in *me*! Well it's gonna stop right *now!*"

I was shocked that Keith was yelling at his doctors—and stunned that he could ignore this new evidence. Finding a nodule was frighteningly significant. I no longer even *considered* stopping here. This *had* to be pursued.

Dr. Barrett took the outburst in stride. He calmly pulled up a chair, sat down beside us, and told Keith he could appreciate how he was feeling. Keith looked past him to the diplomas on the wall, refusing to meet his eyes.

The physician reviewed the important factors of prostate cancer for both of us, emphasizing the high death rate.

"If you were thirty years older, Keith, I might agree with doing nothing but 'watchful waiting,'" Dr. Barrett said, his voice intense. "But not at your age. You're only forty-nine, and you have a lot of years left. I'd feel I'd been negligent if I didn't encourage you to have this biopsy."

Keith turned to face the urologist, his features disclosing no hint of what he was thinking.

"Please reconsider," added Dr. Barrett.

We didn't stay long after that. Keith quickly assured the physician he would think about "everything," and promised to call within the week with his decision.

On the ride home from the Clinic, I was quiet, needing to be alone with my thoughts. This appointment had been incredibly disheartening. The frightening findings—and Keith's strenuous outburst—left me feeling helpless.

But, I reminded myself, he didn't shut the door completely. He did say he would "think about things."

I looked over at Keith, his hands gripping and ungripping the steering wheel, and my heart softened. I loved this man so much, and hated the thought of anything or anyone hurting him.

"It's been a hard two years, hasn't it?" I asked.

"Yeah, it has," Keith answered, exhaling deeply. "It's been a real bear. And it just doesn't stop."

"Are you afraid, Keith?"

Keith turned his head briefly from the road to me, his expression calm now. Then he turned back to the wheel. "I'm not so much afraid as I am…frustrated," he said slowly. "It's like everyone's trying to push me into making decisions that *they* think are the right thing for me to do. And you *know* I don't like that!" The ends of his mouth crimped quickly, in a tight humorless grin.

Yes, I knew that.

Keith went on. "I don't like feeling backed into a corner, Gin. It's like I have no influence over the outcome of this…" He trailed off.

"I'm not used to feeling so out of control."

"I know this has been hard for you, hon," I said, reaching over to rub the back of Keith's neck.

He leaned his head into my hand. Closing his eyes just for a second, he smiled slightly.

We drove on quietly for a few miles before Keith spoke again.

"It's been hard on you too, Gin. I know that. I know there've been times when our arguments have really hurt you, and I'm sorry about that."

Keith paused.

"But there's so much at stake here. If I *do* have cancer, I can't just blindly say yes to something that could leave me powerless. Can you understand that?"

I nodded my head, not so much in agreement, but in recognition of the welcome apology.

For the remainder of the trip, I watched the barren landscape pass by outside my window. The farms of Minnesota looked lifeless in January, encrusted in their snow-bank fortresses, waiting to be rescued by the first warm days of spring.

Tears started to roll down my cheeks, and my heart raced again as I considered the very real possibility of Keith having prostate cancer.

Oh God, please make him say yes to this biopsy, I prayed silently. Or if that can't happen, I added, feeling child-like, make this all just a horrible dream.

The day after the appointment, Beth phoned from her home in Washington State. She could tell I was upset.

"What's wrong, Mom?" she asked in a worried voice.

I broke down immediately. "It's your Dad."

My words rushed out in a wobbly voice. "They're almost positive he has cancer, and he says he won't have a third biopsy! Says he's sick of the whole thing! Then there's treatment. Your father's so afraid of becoming impotent, he'd rather *die* than have surgery! What if he *does* have cancer?" I managed to gasp. "His concern over keeping his sex life is going to kill him!"

There was quiet on the other end of the line as Beth let me cry into the phone.

When my sobs had subsided, she asked, tentatively, "Mom, do you remember the conversation you had with Steven and me when we were teenagers?"

I wasn't sure which "conversation" Beth was referring to.

"The one you had with us about how we should feel about sex," she prompted gently. "It seemed so important to you that we learn to truly appreciate it. You said we should think of sex as a chance to give and receive pleasure through our bodies," Beth continued. "I remember you saying 'Never be ashamed or embarrassed about your sex drive. Treasure it as a beautiful gift.'"

"Do you remember that talk, Mom?"

Of course I remembered that talk almost ten years earlier. I was stunned that Beth, too, remembered it so clearly. Talking to the children like that had been such a turning point in my *own* life.

I had been raised to be a "good girl" where sex was concerned. My conservative, religious parents had instilled in me a belief that sex was wrong before marriage, after which, it became miraculously all right. Consequently, when Keith and I married at the age of 21, I was shy and hesitant in my sexual behavior, and certainly inexperienced.

Keith was different. He was liberal, daring, and anxious to experiment. Keith thought of sex as a natural part of being human, and something we should never hesitate to enjoy. Our two very different views about sex had sometimes caused problems in our marriage. Until the day I had had "that talk" with the children.

It had been such an awakening to hear myself. I'd realized I was parroting Keith's words and attitudes, telling the children what Keith had been telling me for the first seventeen years of our marriage. What a revelation it had been to discover that I had mentally adopted Keith's beliefs, but had never actually put them into practice.

I could always speak frankly with Beth, and was doubly glad right now that our relationship was so open. I answered my daughter.

"Yes, I remember, Beth. As a matter of fact, it was after that talk with you and Steven that I decided to be more open about sex myself."

I thought about how proud I was for doing that. For changing. For being more open to experimenting. For not holding back so much. The process had been slow, and my metamorphosis certainly wasn't complete, but things were definitely better. In the last ten years, our sex life had become much more satisfying to both of us, mostly because I had been willing to change. Sex was more exciting now than it had ever been. And we expected it to only get better.

When I got off the phone, I thought again about how important sex really was in our marriage. For the first time, I felt some empathy for Keith's fears—and hesitantly acknowledged to myself that it might be hard to give up what we now had.

But still. I couldn't go so far as to agree that Keith shouldn't have this biopsy—or surgery if he needed it! Besides, I justified, if he *did* have to have the surgery, there's no way he would become impotent. It would just be too ironic.

In the end, Keith agreed to have a third biopsy. But he agreed *only* with my complete understanding—and that of Dr. Barrett—that this was to be the last. If no cancer was found, Keith would not allow us to go through this stress again.

Two weeks later, the procedure was performed. Cells were extracted and sent to the pathologist. Once again, we were left waiting for the results, wondering if our life would be forever changed. Wondering if we would survive what might follow. Wondering if cancer was already spreading through Keith's body.

We had stopped arguing, at least for the time being. Now we were just holding our breath.

Chapter Two

Our Cancer Nightmare Comes True

On the day we were to get "the news," we tried to keep things as normal as possible. Keith made arrangements to work from home. I attended an early-morning business meeting. Both of us cleared our calendars for 11:00 a.m.—the time Dr. Barrett said he would call.

Unfortunately, my meeting ran over and, despite driving like a bat out of hell, I didn't get home until 11:10. I felt guilty when I walked into Keith's office, thinking I had let him down and not been there for him. But Keith was talking on his business phone. I was instantly relieved. Surely, I thought, the fact that he's back to work means he received good news!

As I walked toward Keith, he casually handed me a piece of paper filled with handwritten notes. At the top of the page was the title "PHONE CALL WITH DR. BARRETT."

I began to read, still anticipating all was well. The words on the page jumped out at me.

Biopsy is positive…adenocarcinoma…left lobe… probably confined…come in next week to discuss options… suggest surgery and taking of pelvic lymph nodes…

I immediately thought I must have misread. If Keith has cancer, *what is he doing* talking on the phone and conducting business as usual?

Yes, I assured myself, I've misread. I scanned the scrap of paper again.

"Biopsy is positive…adenocarcinoma…"

Suddenly I felt faint. I was falling into a dark tunnel, like Alice tumbling down the rabbit hole. Everything in the room began to spin, and familiar objects looked tilted and surreal. I fell clumsily into a chair, and was grateful to hear Keith's voice, as if from a distance.

"I've got to go now. I'll call you back later."

For the next few seconds we stared at each other in silence. When I finally found my voice, I blurted out, "What does this mean?"

The question sounded absurd to me even as I asked it.

Keith's reply was simple: "I have prostate cancer."

I wanted to scream, "NO! Don't *say* that!" and run out of the house—away from this horrible "thing" that had infected our lives. But I couldn't get out of the chair. I felt paralyzed, instantly severed from the thread of hope I had clung to over the last two years. Our cancer nightmare *had* come true.

Despite all the doctors, the gathered reports and the discussions, it was only now becoming a reality for me.

My stomach began to cramp. I could feel the color drain from my face.

Keith reached for my hand and held it gently. His eyes reflected concern. Keith always gets upset when he sees me hurting, and I knew that, despite the overwhelming news, he was more concerned about my feelings right then than his own.

"How do *you* feel about this?" I whispered, dragging my focus back to Keith again.

"I'm numb," he replied in a level tone. "I can't take it all in."

Keith paused. "I guess I knew it all along, but when I heard the words I couldn't believe it. I just stopped feeling."

"How could you go *on*?" I asked incredulous. "Make your phone call and do business?"

"What else was I supposed to do?" Keith answered quietly. "I can't do anything to change this."

For the rest of that day, we tried to work—Keith in his office and me in mine, two floors above. But we couldn't stay apart. We kept "running into one another" in the kitchen, the porch or the den. When we did, we welcomed the embraces that followed. We held on to each other a lot that day, clinging for strength.

Keith asked me to be the one to call the children and my mom. "I know it sounds strange," he said, responding to my puzzled expression, "but having cancer somehow makes me feel ashamed. I just want to crawl in a hole like a hurt animal."

I reached out to hold him, and Keith's voice murmured in my ear: "I don't want to talk to anyone about it right now."

So *I* placed the calls, hating the fact that I would have to speak out loud the awful words that had ricocheted around my head all day.

Beth took the news in her typical stoic manner. "Mom," she told me, "our family can handle anything."

Steven was equally supportive, but more outwardly emotional. Despite the fact that his post-graduate work was entirely focused on cancer research, the diagnosis of his own dad hit him hard. Fighting back tears, he said he'd fly out to be with us anytime we needed him.

The call to Mom was difficult. Hearing of Keith's cancer, I knew, would remind Mom of her own battle with stomach cancer—a topic she tried her best to avoid discussing. It wasn't surprising, therefore, that Mom said little more than to tell us how sorry she was.

We went to bed early that night and instinctively fell into each other's arms. Our love-making was emotional, and afterward we held each other's bodies protectively, trying to ward off the demons in our future.

Sleep was long in coming that night, and when it did finally overtake us, it did little to refresh the soul.

* * *

The next morning, my first waking thought was of cancer.

I looked at Keith, still sleeping, his hair rumpled and his face smooth. "Cancer is eating away at Keith's body," I thought, horrified.

At breakfast, Keith told me he felt "unclean."

We plodded through each day that week, completely unnerved and unsure how to react in the face of the diagnosis. We got through work as best we could, but were always anxious to return to the haven of home each night, where we could be together.

Laptop Notes, January 23, 1995

Tomorrow is my appointment at Mayo to "discuss options".

Still thinking of doing nothing, waiting to see how things develop. Prostate cancer is generally slow-growing. We may have some time.

Not that I want to take risks.

I have a dream of sitting on a porch swing with Gin when we're in our eighties, watching the family around us. I want Duncan to know his Grandpa, to remember that I took him fishing and flying. And Beth and Carew say they are planning a big family. I can't miss that.

But I also can't risk this surgery.

Journal Entry, January 23, 1995

Dear God, please let Keith say yes to the operation. Let him agree to get this cancer out of his body so he can be well again…so we can have our old life back. Now that we know for sure, we <u>have</u> to get rid of it.

This past week has been horrible with all the waiting and worrying...but at the same time it's also been good in a strange sort of way. Keith and I aren't fighting anymore. We're back to being close, realizing how much we mean to each other. And it feels good to be making love and loving again.
Now if he'll only have the surgery, all will be well.

Our appointment with Dr. Barrett took place in his office. Here, there were no examining tables, no intimidating instruments, no charts—only a paper-laden desk, lots of hardcover books neatly arranged in a mahogany bookcase, and three chairs, thoughtfully positioned in a circle.

Dr. Barrett began the meeting by telling us how sorry he was that Keith had cancer. He said that, while he wasn't surprised by the biopsy results, he nevertheless found no joy in "being right." His focus at this point was to help us choose the appropriate course of treatment for Keith's disease.

Dr. Barrett then talked about the characteristics and progression of prostate cancer, and reminded Keith of the seriousness of his condition. Of all the treatments available for prostate cancer, the urologist preferred surgery. This option, he said, offered the greatest possibility for a cure.

To prove his point, Dr. Barrett showed us graphs comparing the life-expectancy results of patients treated for prostate cancer, using either surgery or radiation therapy. The lines on the graphs were identical for almost ten years, then one line dropped slightly while the other remained level. Dr. Barrett noted that the line that stayed level reflected the success of surgery in providing longevity.

Everything about the meeting was pleasing me. Both the circled chairs and Dr. Barrett's caring demeanor were comforting. I liked the way he was handling the situation, and the information he was providing could not have been more convincing.

But still, I was concerned. What comes across as reassuring to me often appears patronizing to Keith. I glanced nervously over at him, trying to decipher how he was receiving Dr. Barrett's presentation. But nothing about his appearance indicated that Keith was either disturbed or resistant. He was sitting with his hands resting easily in his lap, looking relaxed and attentive.

Feeling relieved, I turned my attention back to the explanation of the operation.

Keith listened intently while Dr. Barrett spoke of recovery time and outcome. Only when he paused did Keith ask the question that overshadowed all other input for him: "And what about the possibility of becoming impotent?"

Dr. Barrett readily acknowledged that impotence was an unfortunate risk associated with the operation.

"But," he quickly pointed out, "that risk is low…about 30%[1]. And you're young. The odds are in your favor."

Keith then questioned Dr. Barrett about the nerve-sparing technique. This technique of prostate surgery, pioneered at Johns Hopkins by Dr. Patrick Walsh, was a procedure Keith had read a lot about. He knew it could save many of the nerves required for a man to achieve an erection.

"Do you use this procedure here?" Keith asked.

"I do," the surgeon replied readily. "But you can't assume that the nerve-sparing technique guarantees an escape from impotence. There are other factors besides nerve damage that can affect a man's ability to achieve an erection, such as blood loss and arterial damage. Those causes are almost impossible to predict."

We all sat in silence for a moment.

Dr. Barrett looked at both of us, perhaps realizing that he had hit upon a point of resistance. He leaned close, and concluded with a powerful reassurance.

"Look Keith, if you do become impotent, don't worry. We can easily treat it. These days we have excellent methods for creating erections. We're using a new injectable medication that

---

[1] *This figure has since been the focus of a great deal of controversy, and, depending on sources, can range anywhere from 30% to as high as 80%.*

gives a man an erection just like the natural thing. So don't be concerned."

I was surprised and disappointed when Dr. Barrett ended the meeting by telling us he didn't want Keith to make a decision today.

"Think about it for a week," he suggested, asking that we notify him when a conclusion had been reached.

I gave an inner sigh. Another week without a decision? Another week for the cancer to spread? Why couldn't we just decide *today*?

Neither Keith nor I spoke as we left Dr. Barrett's office and headed across the street for our next appointment—at the Calvary Episcopal Church. The air was crisp and invigorating, and we held hands, skirting patches of dirty city snow on our way to the Tudor-style sanctuary in the middle of the Mayo campus. We were on our way to see Nicklas Mezacapa, an Episcopalian priest and a member of the Prostate Cancer Support Group in Rochester. Dr. Barrett had recommended we talk to Nick, a man around Keith's age who had survived prostate cancer thanks to the same surgery he wanted us to consider.

Keith's willingness to accept this suggestion had been only mildly surprising to me. In the week following the cancer diagnosis, the focus of our conversations about surgery had shifted. Keith had moved from stating that he wouldn't even consider surgery to telling me he was "still exploring all possibilities" and assimilating facts.

I understood this shift. With a confirmed diagnosis, death had instantly moved from being an abstract possibility to an ominous reality. Now both of us thought of little else.

Father Nick met us in his rectory with a warm handshake and an easy smile. He seemed pleased to share his experiences, and immediately made us feel comfortable, pouring us a cup of tea as he began.

Father Nick had been diagnosed with prostate cancer at the age of thirty-nine, and had elected to have a prostatectomy (prostate surgery in which the prostate gland is removed). He told us it had now been seven years since his operation and, in his experience at least, it had been a blessing. He was still disease-free and doing great.

When Keith asked him if "doing great" meant "great in all areas," Father Nick grinned coyly and nodded.

"Like many Episcopalian priests, I'm married," he volunteered. "And I can assure you that I function just like I did before the surgery. No problems whatsoever."

As we walked back to the Clinic from Father Nick's parish, Keith unexpectedly took my hand, and, like a happy schoolboy, began swinging it back and forth.

"That was really good for me to hear," he said as we crossed the street.

I looked up. Keith was grinning that wonderful half smile of his. It felt so good to be seeing that smile again! I skipped a step, and swung his hand higher.

Impulsively, Keith turned and gave me a quick kiss, before opening the door to the Clinic.

Our final appointment that day was with Dr. Phyliky. Our family doctor for over seven years, Dr. Phyliky wanted to meet with us to discuss any concerns we might still have.

The cold examination room warmed instantly upon Dr. Phyliky's arrival. He was a small-framed man with graying temples. His soft-spoken, gentle manner was calming, and his compassion sincere. Both of us trusted him completely.

Dr. Phyliky began by asking Keith what he had learned from Dr. Barrett and Nick, and how he was now feeling about his situation.

Keith quickly summarized the two earlier meetings. Then he very casually concluded: "…and I've made up my mind to go ahead with the surgery."

I was dumbstruck! Keith had decided to have the surgery! I couldn't believe it! It was all I could do to stay put in my chair. I wanted to leap up and smother him with kisses. To laugh. Shout for joy. Cry with relief.

I tried to compose myself, and managed to stay seated, but, inside, I was nearly bursting.

Dr. Phyliky nodded and smiled approvingly.

"Now that you've made up your mind about treatment, Keith, I feel I can comment on your decision," he noted. "I'm very pleased that you've elected to have surgery. Like Dr. Barrett, I feel it gives you the greatest possibility for a cure."

He cleared his throat before continuing.

"I must tell you that my father just recently died of prostate cancer, and I was with him until the end."

Once again that day, we were both silent.

"Prostate cancer kills many men," Dr. Phyliky stated soberly. "And believe me, it's not a good way to die."

Journal Entry, January 24, 1995

I am SO surprised when Keith said he'd decided to have the surgery!

Rule follower that I am, I expected to be waiting out a horrible week "thinking it over" like Dr. Barrett asked. But then Keith just went with his gut and decided!

For the first time in <u>days</u> I feel like I can take a deep breath.

Now everything is going to be alright.

The kids are happy too. Steven has been a big help during all this, giving us information and talking to fellow researchers and doctors at Johns Hopkins. He says he'll come home to be with me during the operation, and I'm really glad. I sure could use his company.

Keith's going to have surgery! Prayers are indeed answered!

January 25, 1995

TO ALL EMPLOYEES:

In an effort to dispel any rumors you may have heard recently, I would like to share some facts with you about my personal health.

An elevated PSA (Prostate Specific Antigen) test over the past three years has driven the need for me to have annual biopsies. Unfortunately, my most recent biopsy has turned up positive for adenocarcinoma (cancer of the prostate gland).

I am fortunate that this was found in the earliest stage detectable, and that the prognosis is very good. Although prostate cancer is the number two cause of death in men, when found early, treatment is quite successful. Remission is in the 90+% category. Side effects are generally minimal today.

I am scheduled to undergo surgery 2-4-1995 at Saint Mary's in Rochester. This is considered major surgery and I am expected to stay in the hospital for six days, and away from work from three to six weeks afterward.

I will be actively involved with current projects until 1-30-1995. Joyce and I are adjusting schedules accordingly.

Should you have any questions about my schedule, projects, or condition, please stop by. I am very open about the subject and willing to explain to whatever detail you may want.

I want you to know this information from me, as you may be hearing comments from those inside the company, and possibly from the community at large. I'd rather you know the facts.

Thanks for your support.

Keith Laken

Laptop Notes, January 28, 1995

When I sent out my memo, I didn't expect much response. But saying I was willing to answer questions must have opened the floodgates.

For two days I haven't gotten any work done. People have been in my office constantly, some wishing me well, others with questions.

The amazing thing was how many told me about their fathers, brothers, and uncles who had prostate cancer, and how worried they were about them. Some people hugged me. Some even cried.

It was really embarrassing. I didn't know people cared so much.

CHAPTER THREE

Keith Goes Under the Knife

Laptop Notes, February 3, 1995
Tomorrow I go under the knife. My first operation, and I'm really nervous.
I don't like putting my life in someone else's hands, but that's what has to be done. Now I just want to get the whole thing over with.
It was a tough decision to have this surgery, but I won't second guess myself. I never do.

Journal Entry, February 3, 1995
Tomorrow Keith has his surgery. God, I'm scared. I know he needs this operation, but I'm still so worried. Something could go wrong.
I'll be glad when it's all over...the stress is really getting to me.
Tonight Keith wanted to make love "for old-times sake." I just went through the motions. I couldn't concentrate. I really don't know how Keith can do it. How he can have a climax at a

time like this??? He can just put things out of his mind and go on. I wish I could be like that.

Keith's been so concerned about being impotent, I'm sure that's why he wanted to make love tonight. But I just couldn't get into it.

It's not <u>*important*</u> *to me that we have sex. I don't care about that.*

I JUST WANT KEITH TO LIVE.

On February 4, 1995, Keith kissed me good-bye before technicians wheeled him from his hospital room. I had tears in my eyes, and my knees felt weak. Steven walked beside me as we headed downstairs toward the surgery waiting area—the same room I had waited in during Mom's operation three years earlier. Mom was still fighting her cancer, and I shuddered at the thought that this disease was attacking those I held dearest.

The small room was filled with people sitting in clusters, talking in whispers. We found a place to sit as far away as possible from anyone else. Like the others in the room, we just wanted to be alone.

Steven and I sat silently for a long time. Then I tried to busy myself.

I attempted a crossword puzzle, but quickly put it down. I picked up a magazine, but found nothing interesting. I got a cup of coffee, but couldn't drink it.

All I could think about was Keith, lying on the operating table, *being cut open.* I prayed for many things: that Keith would recover; that the cancer hadn't spread; that I wouldn't leave the hospital a widow.

I tried to calm my fears by reminding myself that we were in one of the best medical facilities in the world, and that people don't die from surgery anymore. That Keith was young.

But my self-talk wasn't very convincing.

Steven was a godsend. He was only 24, but he wisely knew exactly how long to let me stew before speaking to me, and then he was understanding and consoling. He held my hand and rubbed my shoulders.

I thought about what a beautiful person Steven was: such a nice blend of analytical scientist and humanistic healer. We were so proud of him, working on his Ph.D. in cancer research. How ironic that he was here, waiting for his own dad to come out of cancer surgery.

After about three hours, the "communication nurse" called my name.

"The operation is over," she said, her face offering no clues. "Your husband is in recovery. You'll be able to see him soon."

I had been praying to hear these words, yet even as the nurse said them, they did little to allay my fears. Until I actually saw Keith, it would impossible for me to relax.

When I did see him, however, I was shocked. He looked so vulnerable—so pale and fragile in his anesthetic induced unconsciousness. I immediately tried to reassure myself: At least he's still alive.

Everything about that day was arduous. Keith was restless and in a great deal of pain, and I felt helpless. There was little I could do to comfort him.

"Hang in there, Mom," Steven reminded me. "In a way, today's probably harder on you than Dad. He won't remember most of it."

The next morning, Steven and I went back to the hospital early. We wanted to be sure to be there when Dr. Barrett made his morning rounds. This was the day we would all hear the pathology report.

"You folks have dodged a bullet," Dr. Barrett began, when he saw us sitting with Keith. "The tumor was much larger than we thought. It encompassed about 30 percent of the prostate. It was also more aggressive than we suspected. The pathologist rated it a Grade 3+4 out of 10 on the Gleason Scale."

We all knew this was a dangerous-size tumor, and the shock must have registered on our faces.

Dr. Barrett continued in an optimistic tone. "Fortunately the tumor was confined to the prostate, and hadn't invaded any surrounding tissue. But it certainly needed to come out—and it looks like we got it just in time."

Keith's hospital recovery went well, and three days after his operation they told us he would be discharged the next day. He would come home with a catheter inserted in his bladder and a drainage bag strapped to his leg—standard procedure for prostatectomy patients. In three weeks, the catheter would be removed. Then, if all went well, Keith would experience only a short period of incontinence.

Recovery from the possibility of permanent impotence would be the final stage of the healing process. That recovery, we had learned, could take two years or more.

Laptop Notes, February 7, 1995
    Surgery's over. What a relief.
    Overall it wasn't as bad as I thought it'd be.
    My penis, on the other hand! The first time I got a look at it, I couldn't believe it. It's wider than it is long! Huge, swollen, and all black and blue.
    They put this big catheter in it. How it doesn't hurt I don't know. The nurse said when it comes out I'll be incontinent for awhile.
    That kind of scares me.
    Still, I'm glad to be going home with Gin. She's been by my side this whole time. I couldn't have gotten through this without her.
    She really keeps me going.

Journal Entry, February 7, 1995

It will be so good to have Keith home where I can take care of him. I find it hard seeing him in the hospital. He looks so wounded.

I brought him his laptop and some magazines and books, since he asked for them. I don't think he knows how to just rest. Maybe when he's home and comfortable...

I hate seeing him wear that leg bag. As much as I don't like to admit it, I sometimes think about how terrible it would be if he were permanently incontinent. That would really be awful.

We're so lucky Keith is young and healthy.

When Keith arrived home from the hospital we spent most of the day getting him settled. I unpacked his suitcase, made up a day bed on the sofa in the family room, and, together, we nervously fumbled with catheter cleaning and changing.

"I want to help you with that," I told Keith as he started to unstrap his leg bag.

"No I can do it by myself. That's all right."

"No, please! I want to help," I offered. "Let's do it together. While you're putting on the new bag, I'll clean the old one."

Turning aside, I mumbled, "Now what did Nancy say about the proportion of vinegar to water?"

"Gin, let me *do* it!" Keith said, annoyed, grabbing for the vinegar jar.

I instinctively pulled back, and the acidic smell of vinegar filled the bathroom as the bottle slipped from my hand, splashing onto the tile floor.

Keith looked at me with an expression of disgust, and we both grabbed towels. We were working furiously to sop up the liquid, but we made little headway; the more we wiped, the more seemed to appear.

Frustrated with our lack of progress, we sat back and looked around the room, then at each other. In our haste to clean up the vinegar puddle, Keith had forgotten to clamp his catheter tubing. And the liquid we were now wiping was not vinegar, but urine—pouring from his leg bag!

In desperation, Keith attempted to squeeze the spigot on the wet, slippery bag. After four tries, he was finally able to contain the flood.

When all was under control, we sat back once more and looked at ourselves. What a prize we both were! We began to smirk at each other, then to chuckle. Finally we laughed out loud —heads thrown back, arms around our stomachs. When we were able to contain ourselves, Keith reached over to touch my shoulder.

"I'm sorry for getting grumpy, Gin. Thanks for all your help," he said warmly. "I really couldn't have done this without you."

"No problem, hon, really. Anytime you need me, I'll be right here," I replied, giving him a kiss.

It was so good to be home and to be together.

The catheter incident definitely helped relieve some of our first-day-home-together tension, but not all of it. That night it surfaced again as we debated about sleeping together.

Keith was concerned that I might unintentionally hurt him during the night, by draping a leg over him or kicking him. But we had never slept apart, other than when one of us traveled, and we didn't really want to start now. So, despite his worries, we decided to take the risk.

The next morning when we awoke in each other's arms, we knew we'd made the right decision. We kissed each other good morning, breathed a sigh of relief, and faced the second day of Keith's return home in a much more relaxed frame of mind.

The experience of being together at home all day long with no commitments felt like a rare gift to us. We hardly ever had "home time" like this together during the week.

There was still this incontinence issue that might be a problem, but there was no point in worrying about that for at least the next three weeks. Right then, we wanted to savor our time together.

On that first full day at home, we spent the morning doing routine tasks. In the afternoon, we relaxed on the sofa in the family room in front of a warm fire. Soon we began to recount our individual feelings about the past few days, weeks, and months.

We both cried as we relived the fears and anxieties that had plagued our lives for so long.

When we were done, we felt cleansed and ready to move on.

"Gin, it meant so much to me to have you there when I woke up this morning," Keith said, stroking my hair.

We were cozy in our nest, while February slushed and dripped outside the window. "Having you by my side through all this is helping me stay positive."

"Oh, Keith, I wouldn't have been anywhere else *but* by your side. I love you."

Keith carefully stretched his legs, and I sat up straight to look at him properly.

"Our marriage is so important to me," he stated, looking deeply into my eyes. "*You're* so important to me. You've always given so much of yourself to me and the kids. I wouldn't be where I am today if I didn't have you."

It was so good to hear Keith reaffirm our marriage and our love, which had been battered during the stress of the last two years.

I felt the same way.

"You've made me a better person, too," I said, hugging him. "You've taught me so much about life and love. Being married to you has been the best part of my life."

I smiled, sure that we had made it through some of our darkest hours. "We've become a good team, haven't we?"

"Yep," he agreed. "Together we can survive anything."

* * *

Throughout the remainder of that day we barely left each other's side. We touched and hugged continually. Keith's physical vulnerability made me feel all the more tender toward him.

By evening, our hugging had progressed to passionate kissing, and we began to touch each other in delight. I was surprised to realize what was happening—I was becoming aroused.

I was torn. I knew we couldn't make love, but I was really enjoying the teasing and intimacy at the same time.

Finally, I told Keith, breathless, "We'd better stop. I'm getting really turned on! And I don't want to end up being frustrated and spoil this perfect day..."

Keith smiled and whispered in my ear. "Let's go to bed. I'm going to make you feel good."

"What are you thinking?" I protested.

"Just leave it up to me," he said, kissing my neck. "Don't worry about anything. I can *do* this."

Keith took my hand and led me upstairs.

Nervous at first, a little scared and wary, I finally couldn't resist any longer. I had had an emotional, loving day with the man I adored, and now I wanted Keith so badly.

As I lay naked on the bed, not knowing what to expect, Keith knelt on the floor beside me. He resumed kissing and caressing me. He used our vibrator to increase my desire. And when I could stand it no longer, his fingers brought me to orgasm.

At the very peak of my climax, I started to cry, then to sob. I was overwhelmed.

Here was Keith, five days from surgery, with a catheter in his penis, giving me such physical pleasure and release. It was the most selfless act I could imagine.

His love for me was humbling.

I knew I was the luckiest woman in the world!

Laptop Notes, February 10, 1995
    It was great to be able to make Gin so happy last night! Nothing makes me feel as good

32

as when I can get her aroused. When I know she wants me and I can drive her wild.

Gin didn't hold back, either, which was great. She let me do whatever I wanted, and I totally satisfied her.

Being her lover is one of the greatest pleasures in my life.

Journal Entry, February 10, 1995

Last night was the most romantic and beautiful night of my life! I've never felt so adored! I'll never, ever forget it.

This experience was so different from our usual. We've never made love when I was the only one to have an orgasm.

Before last night, if Keith had suggested masturbating me, I would have refused. I guess I always thought married couples wouldn't need to do that kind of thing. But last night, everything was different...what we did seemed so natural.

I can only think of the whole experience as one of complete devotion.

To this day, Keith and I both refer to our lovemaking on that glorious night as one of the ultimate sexual expressions of love in our marriage. The intensity of our love-making reflected a new appreciation for the fragility of life—and the joy of being survivors.

Together, we had celebrated life, love and our marriage.

We were full of hope then, and were able to look past the recovery period, toward future nights of fulfillment. Everything was behind us, we thought.

It was probably a blessing, on that perfect night, that we didn't know our celebration would continue for only a few short months. Then our relationship would once again be threatened.

This time the threat would not be to Keith's life, but rather to his sense of manliness. And, for him, that would be almost as bad.

Looking Back
I Wish I Hadn't Said That to Keith

Today, I shudder when I look back at what I said to Keith when he initially was concerned about becoming impotent.

Words that were meant to reassure ended up discounting his feelings. And while my intention was always to comfort Keith, instead I was demeaning—not only to him, but to myself and to our relationship as well.

When I said I wouldn't miss having sex, I was certain I was speaking the truth—that just having Keith alive and well would more than make up for not having intercourse. But I was wrong. My basic sexual drive was stronger than I had anticipated. Within days of Keith's surgery, I found myself longing to make love with him again. And this desire never abated. In fact, the strength of it surprised me. Obviously, I had underestimated the importance sex played in my physical well-being.

I had similarly undervalued the delicate interweaving of sex and intimacy in our marriage. While I had always respected the role sexual intimacy played in a committed relationship, what I didn't appreciate was how often Keith and I had, throughout our 27 years of marriage, made love after experiencing a significant emotional event. Whether it was in happiness or in sorrow, the act of sharing our bodies with each other had always made me feel closer to Keith. And this was something I hadn't fully acknowledged when I so glibly stated "it won't matter if we don't have sex anymore."

These words were most demeaning, however, to Keith. In the early days of our impotency debates, I stopped listening when Keith would try to explain how interconnected his sexual performance was to his sense of *being*, his sense of competence and his self-image. I discounted his statement that it was important to him to be able to satisfy me. I'm ashamed to say that I only really started to listen to these feelings when I became fearful for the future of our marriage.

Today, when I hear women trying to comfort their partners with the same phrases I used, I cringe. I want to tell them: "You're wrong when you say you won't miss making love to your man, because you will. And please honor him by telling him so."

I want to encourage these compassionate women, who mean so well, to learn from my mistakes. Accept your partner's fears as normal, not just as "male vanity." Tell your soul mate that his loss is a loss to you as well.

If I could do it all over again, knowing what I know now, I think I would express myself this way:

"Keith, if you become impotent, I understand that things will change in our sexual relationship, and that we will have to significantly alter the way we make love. That's frightening, but I know we can get through it. Even though we don't really know what those changes might be right now, I'm committed to doing whatever is necessary to keep our sex life alive. In return, I'll depend on you to remain a lover to me in whatever way is possible. I'm confident that we can continue to make each other happy and satisfied in ways we'll be able to discover—together."

CHAPTER FOUR

You Can't Have An Orgasm
Without An Erection...Can You?

During the first few weeks of his recovery, Keith was uncomfortable, tired, and pretty content to stay around the house and let me take care of him. I enjoyed the chance to pamper him a little; it satisfied my nurturing spirit. I brought him his lunch on a tray, fluffed his pillows and made sure he took his medications on time.

Keith had initially protested my taking six weeks off from my consulting business to tend to him, saying it was "totally unnecessary." But after the first couple of days home, he admitted he was glad I was there.

"We haven't had the chance to spend this much time together all at once in our entire marriage," he told me. "And I like it!"

At the end of the third week, Keith had his catheter removed. He was, just as we had been forewarned, incontinent.

We had expected this, but oh the reality!

Keith was extremely embarrassed over having no bladder control, and humiliated by having to wear adult diapers.

For three weeks he agonized over going back to work. What if someone could tell he was wearing one? What if it leaked?

As the time drew nearer, Keith performed numerous dress rehearsals in anticipation of that first day back. He put on his dress pants, tucked in his shirt, and had me check him out.

"Be honest," he would say. "Can you see anything?"

I always assured him, truthfully, that he was fine. "No one will know anything is different, hon."

The first day of his seventh week post-surgery, Keith went back to work. He sat behind his desk that first morning, still apprehensive about what people would think. But the welcome he received from his co-workers quickly helped lessen his fears. Almost everyone in the plant made a point to stop by his office and tell him how much they'd missed him. Many gave him hugs. Some brought gifts of food. Keith was very moved, and, by the end of that day, much of his anxiety had subsided.

Keith's incontinence lasted for about two months after the catheter was removed, which was considered remarkably short (but felt remarkably long to him). We attributed his speedy recovery to two factors. First, Keith had faithfully performed the recommended bladder-strengthening exercises every day. Second, he was only 49, which we thought had the most significant impact.

In fact, Keith's entire recovery from surgery was amazingly quick and easy. Because of this, we took it for granted that his *whole* recovery would progress rapidly as well. We happily assumed that, any day, Keith would experience a quick and total return to sexual functioning.

No such luck.

As the days went by, we saw no improvement at all. No signs of healing or recovery. Nothing.

And, after three months, our optimism started to waver.

Laptop Notes, May 1, 1995

Three months since my surgery. Three months without sex.

I've never gone this long before, and I don't want to go much longer. I should be seeing some sign by now!

At first I wasn't thinking about sex much. Too preoccupied with peeing all the time. But this last month I've been thinking about it a lot. And nothing is happening. I've tried to get it hard myself but it's no use.

Shit! How can I do anything when I'm like this? I can't come on to Gin when I can't even get a hard-on. It would be too humiliating.

Journal Entry, May 3, 1995

We haven't made love again since that first night home from the hospital. But that's all right, I can wait.

Keith's getting restless, though. A few times he's hinted at masturbating me again, but I've put him off. I want to wait until he can enjoy himself too.

I've thought of initiating something, but I'm kind of worried about hurting him...laying on his incision...making him strain...

Anyway, it shouldn't be too much longer before we see some signs of healing.

In early May, we went together to Mayo for Keith's three-month check up. Dr. Barrett was pleased with his progress and was very reassuring.

"Keith, you seem to be doing great. Your incision's healing nicely, and the fact that you're no longer incontinent is very encouraging."

"Of course," Dr. Barrett noted, "the best news is that your PSA is non-detectable."

He explained again the importance of this test in the ongoing monitoring of prostate cancer. The PSA would show whether all the cancer had been removed, and, in the future, whether it was recurring.

"Everything looks great," he concluded.

Then Dr. Barrett asked the standard doctor phrase: "Do you have any questions?"

Keith sat taller in his chair. "Only one," he said squaring his shoulders. "When can I start having sex again?"

Dr. Barrett seemed genuinely pleased with Keith's query.

"Whenever you feel up to it," he replied, making a note in the chart. Almost as an afterthought, he added, "And you *do* know you can experience an orgasm without having an erection, don't you?"

Keith nodded confidently. "Sure."

After making a few more notes in Keith's chart, and checking one more time to make sure he had answered all our questions, Dr. Barrett ended the meeting by asking Keith to return in three months for another PSA check.

As we headed down the long corridor leading from the examination room to the exit, I tugged at Keith's hand, trying my best to hurry him along. I was anxious to find a place we could be alone, so I could press him for answers to the many questions *I* now had.

It seemed to take forever for us to round the corner of the registration desk, pass in front of the sober-looking patients in the waiting room, and arrive at the large lobby in front of the elevators. To my relief, the area was deserted.

I put my hand in front of the button, preventing Keith from pressing it. "Wait a minute before you call the elevator," I started, "I have to talk to you first."

Keith looked confused, then concerned. "Okay, what about?"

I stepped back slightly from the elevator doors, pulling Keith gently with me. Leaning close, I spoke in whispers, even though no one else was around.

"Hon, what made you ask Dr. Barrett about having sex?" I asked expectantly. "Has something happened to make you think you're ready?"

Keith looked slightly sheepish. "Well no… The question I had wasn't really whether it was all *right* for us to have sex, but when we could expect it to be *possible*. I mean, how much longer is it going to take 'til I see some signs of life?" Keith glanced downward, shuffling his feet.

"Oh. Well, he obviously didn't answer *that* question. So I guess we still don't know if you're on track or not."

I took one more step backward, my back now touching the wall, and quickly scanned the area one more time for strangers. Reassured that we were still alone, I nevertheless waved Keith closer.

I stood on my toes, reaching up to put my lips right next to his ear.

"Well, then…how about this 'orgasm without an erection' idea? Did you know you could do that?"

Keith blushed, and turned his head away from my whisper.

"I've never heard of such a thing, Gin," he began, stepping back and speaking in a normal tone. "I don't know where this guy's coming from!"

Then he lowered his voice again. "You *can't* have sex without getting an erection. That's where your desire comes from. I don't know why he said that."

"But Keith," I pushed, not willing to be put off, "Dr. Barrett must know what he's talking about. He's a doctor."

I was a little annoyed with Keith. Why hadn't he said anything during the meeting if he'd found the comment so bogus?

"So why didn't you *ask* him about it?" I persisted. "I thought this was something you knew but just never said anything to *me* about."

Keith glanced up the hallway, and then back at me. He, too, was now obviously annoyed.

"Look, I'm *not* going to talk to *Dr. Barrett* about how to have sex! I know how it works! He doesn't have to give me a lesson, for God's sake!"

Keith's mouth formed a thin line as he moved toward the elevator button and pressed it three times in quick succession.

"Either it works or it doesn't, Gin, OK? And if it doesn't, you don't just chit chat about it."

Once again, I just didn't get it. Here was something *important* for us to know—something that might help us have sex again—and Keith wouldn't even talk to his own *doctor* about it?

Feeling pressured to end our conversation before the elevator arrived, I cocked my head and tried to coerce. "Come on, hon. How about calling him in the morning and asking him to tell us more? Please?"

Keith looked at me with a mixture of astonishment and frustration. "Are you *kidding*? There's no way I'm going to call him and talk to him about having an orgasm!"

A few days after our appointment, Steven phoned and asked if we could arrange to take some time off and bring him a few things he'd left at home. Keith and I jumped at the chance.

We always enjoy spending time with Steven, and our opportunities to do so were limited because of the intensity of his grad-school studies. Taking advantage of this opening in his schedule would provide a welcome opportunity to see him. Besides, we both liked Baltimore, and spring was a beautiful time of the year to travel.

I planned our itinerary with eager anticipation. Not only was it going to be good to get away and have a change of scenery, but I had high hopes that the trip would provide an opportunity for us to be intimate again. Trips, and especially hotel rooms, had always been aphrodisiacs for Keith and me, and many of our most memorable lovemaking experiences took place in these "foreign bedrooms." When we were away, we relaxed, using the freedom from day-to-day responsibilities to concentrate on what gave us the most pleasure, which had always included great sex.

Journal Entry, May 5, 1995

I've made up my mind I'm going to try to end our abstinence on this trip. I'm going to test Dr. Barrett's "orgasm without erection" idea. Keith isn't doing anything about initiating sex, and I don't think it's good for us to go any longer without it.

I feel a little shy, though. I've never been very good about taking the lead role. I've always let Keith do that. But now things are different. I have to do something. I'm thinking of it kind of like doing more nursing...the final stage of helping Keith get better. I'm sure once he realizes he can have orgasms again, his doubts about being sexually capable will disappear, and he'll relax and feel good about himself. And once <u>that</u> happens, his erections will quickly follow.

The only question is whether this will work. What if it doesn't?

I can't think about that right now. I've got to do this and help Keith get back to normal.

The first day of our car trip was perfect. The spring flowers were in full bloom and the weather was balmy. Keith and I were in good spirits, and we chatted away as the road and the hours sped by.

We spent our first night in Indiana, with my big brother Rodger and sister-in-law Sue. After one of Sue's famous chicken-and-dumpling dinners, we played cards, all the while telling jokes and reminiscing happily together. Visiting like this, as we'd done so many times in the past, helped reinforce the feeling that life was going to return to normal.

The next morning we left late, did some sightseeing, and stopped, early in the afternoon, in Columbus, Ohio.

We checked in at a big hotel with a broad circular drive. The lobby was expansive and nicely decorated. Four oval windows reflected the sun off of a nearby lake where ducks swam in pairs; dark leather chairs were positioned invitingly in front of a large brick fireplace.

When we reached our room, it was equally well furnished, and it, too, overlooked the lake. We unpacked our bags, feeling pleased with the whole trip so far.

"Let's take a quick swim before we change for dinner," I suggested, coming across my swimsuit.

"I sure could use the exercise," Keith nodded.

The hotel pool was located near the lobby, in a quiet area off by itself. No one else was around, so we had the place to ourselves.

The water was soothingly warm.

At first Keith and I swam independently, letting the tightness dissolve from our car-locked joints. Then, as if drawn by invisible magnets, we slowly drifted toward one another.

We touched lightly. Kissed softly. The weightlessness of our bodies felt wonderful.

We played in the pool for a long time, teasing and seducing one another with our glances.

When we finally returned to our room, we stripped from our bathing suits and immediately began to explore each other's bodies.

"Let's skip dinner," I urged.

Keith eagerly agreed.

We moved to the bed. I started kissing Keith on his chest, arms, and legs.

"I want you to come," I whispered, kissing Keith's ear and moving slightly to nibble the lobe.

Keith's body tensed instantly, and he pulled away from me. "No. I'm really sorry, Gin, but I can't," he protested. "Let me do something for *you*."

I stroked him reassuringly.

"Not this time, hon. I want to see if I can help *you* have an orgasm."

I pushed Keith lightly back onto his pillow. "Just try to relax," I coaxed. "Enjoy yourself. And don't worry about anything."

Keith lay unnaturally still.

"And if nothing happens, so what?" I cajoled. "We've still had a good time, right?"

I resumed kissing him, but Keith remained tense and unsure.

Then I began to perform oral sex, certain that this form of stimulation would guarantee some success. As the minutes ticked by, I tried all the things that usually turned Keith on, yet his penis remained flaccid.

Then, just when my determination began to wane and I was about ready to give up, I noticed a slight increase in Keith's breathing. Encouraged, I continued. Yes, Keith *was* getting aroused—even though his penis stayed soft.

I stopped briefly to kiss his body; then I returned to his groin. Once again, Keith's breathing quickened.

I persisted.

In a few minutes, Keith had an orgasm—his first in almost four months.

As the waves of passion subsided, Keith reached for me and encircled me with his arms. Speechless, we held each other close. When we finally pulled back to kiss, the tears on our cheeks mingled.

"Thank you, thank you," Keith uttered emotionally, squeezing me tight. "I was so afraid I'd lost all feeling—that I was sexually dead. But you've brought me back to life."

"Oh hon, I'm so glad it worked!"

I moved off Keith's chest and lay next to him. "Was it really good for you?"

"Yes, it was *really good* Gin. You were great!" Keith said, endearingly. "And next time, I want you to come too."

I smiled, pleased, and snuggled closer.

"So it felt the same even without an erection?" I asked curiously.

Keith played with my hair, thinking. "It was different, especially to begin with. It took me so long to get turned on. But once I got excited, it was pretty much the same."

He paused, then added pensively, "But it *was* strange. Even though I knew I wasn't going to ejaculate, when it didn't happen, it felt a little weird."

Keith stopped stroking my hair, keeping his hand on my head. He looked out the window at the late-afternoon sun on the lake.

"But I'm not dead...thank God."

I sighed in contentment, and put my hand on Keith's cheek. "Oh babe, I just know everything's going to be okay from now on."

Simultaneous oral sex (the "sixty-nine" position) allowed Keith and me to make love often during the remainder of that trip; and each time we did, it was like experiencing our own intimate spring.

Although Keith was unable to achieve an erection, we were awed by the awakening of his body—and rejuvenated by the fact that we were once again enjoying sex. Our hope and optimism came rushing back. We both assumed that Keith's ability to experience orgasm was an omen of what was to follow.

"It won't be long now until everything is working again," we assured one another. "Probably within a few days, we'll be seeing signs of life."

For the remainder of that trip, however, we focused on the present, because it was totally satisfying to us. We were happy again. Keith was getting better.

And we were making love!

Looking Back
Keith, on being informed...

Back in the early '90s, when I first tried to get information about prostate cancer and possible impotence, the Internet was just beginning to be used regularly. There wasn't much information available, and what was available was generally based on research and studies that were done on men much older than me. To men *my* age, the information didn't seem very relevant.

Today, all that has changed. The Internet is filled with up-to-date, accurate and even first-hand information on both prostate cancer and impotence. (See the Resources section in the back of this book.)

Yet, although information is so readily accessible, the medical community continues to state that only about 10% of the estimated 30 million men who suffer from erectile dysfunction actually seek treatment. Why?

Speaking from experience (after all, I didn't even want to question Dr. Barrett about the "orgasm without erection" idea when he brought it up!), I can say that I think the issues *surrounding* impotence are as complex as the medical condition itself.

First of all, this experience is uncharted territory for most of us men. Generally speaking, we usually possess very little knowledge about how our bodies actually work, and are even less informed about how and why we do or don't get an erection. We've heard no talk from other guys about what they did when they "couldn't get it up anymore," and therefore have little knowledge about where to go or what to do for help when it happens to us.

And of course, we're embarrassed. Our sex lives are not something most of us are comfortable talking about (other than maybe during those teenage years in the locker room), and there's a certain feeling of being labeled as weak or ineffective. The feeling is not unlike the shame and embarrassment that a person feels when confronted with alcoholism or mental illness. Despite all the publicity and education we've heard about these conditions, people are usually still hesitant to admit suffering from them— even to a doctor.

Finally, I think many men suffer from erectile dysfunction as a result of a more slowly occurring event than what I experienced, and they may be willing to actually "forget" how good sex and desire can be. When impotence happens gradually, and over a long period of time, perhaps you can talk yourself into just accepting "how life is now." You compensate in other ways— like getting interested in the computer or a hobby—to make up for what you think is no longer available to you. And you neglect the effort of regaining your sexual performance.

Initially, I, too, wasn't very aggressive in pursuing treatment for myself, probably for all of the reasons I've stated above. Fortunately, however, I was able to get beyond these hurdles before I almost allowed myself to be cheated out of the pleasure of sex—permanently.

And I'm so glad I persevered. I believe all of us deserve to enjoy our lives as fully as possible, and I suspect one of our biggest handicaps to doing so is our own self-judgment.

CHAPTER FIVE

Oral-Sex Shock:
From Honeymoon to Holding Pattern

With lovemaking back in our life, Keith and I were as happy as honeymooners. We called each other four, five, six times a day—just to say "hi." We held hands everywhere we went, played footsie during dinner and sent flowers with love notes attached.

Abstinence had been hard on us. Never before had we gone so long without making love. Even after childbirth, we had barely waited the recommended six weeks' "healing time," and the same had been true after my back surgery and partial hysterectomy.

Four months without sex made me begin to appreciate the integral role sex played in our marriage. Making love was what we did to reconnect when things weren't going well—and how we celebrated when they were. Without sex, we had felt isolated from each other. Nothing seemed to fit together properly, and we had been getting testy with each other.

Now that we were being intimate again, life seemed to easily fall back into place.

"We can wait for healing more easily now," we said to each other confidently, "now that we're making love again."

We began to focus on aspects of our life that had been put on hold. Keith resumed flying, I finished a baby quilt. We started walking again. Walking had always been one of our favorite activities, both for the exercise and for the sharing. Our frequent path walked us through our orchard, into the woods, down to the creek.

During our walks, we talked about anything that came to mind. The topics were as diverse as the countryside we covered: work, politics, religion, food, prejudice, science, you name it.

On one of our walks in early June, we spent most of our time catching up on work and family news. Keith told me about the frustrations he was feeling in starting up an R&D facility for his company. I shared stories of my consulting clients. We talked about how we admired Mom's courage and determination in dealing with her stomach cancer, but questioned how much longer she could continue to live alone in her Florida condo.

Finally, we moved to our favorite topic of conversation —our children and grandbaby.

Duncan was pulling himself up on furniture and taking a few steps. Beth and Carew were making steady progress on their home renovations. Steven's research project on colon cancer was producing interesting results, and it seemed likely that his group would soon announce a breakthrough. At the same time, he told me things were now "serious" with his girlfriend, Haley.

"We're so lucky to have such a good relationship with the kids," I reminded Keith as we stepped over a fallen log. "It's something we always hoped would happen: staying close to them as they became adults. And now it *has* happened."

"Well, a big reason for that is because we've worked at it," Keith replied, putting his arm around me. "Especially you, Gin. Ever since they went away to school you've talked to them practically every day. That's why you always know what issues they're struggling with. You're the one they always look to for advice."

"The kids rely on you, too, hon," I said, protesting. "They always come to you for the really *serious* things… financial stuff, career decisions. Steven, especially, always asks your opinion."

Our walk was over and we were almost back at the house. The evening air was warm, with the sunset coloring the sky, and we just weren't ready to leave the serene outdoor world yet. So we sat on the porch swing and cuddled.

"You know Keith, it's really remarkable how open we've become with the kids over the past few years," I commented, my eyes on the reddening horizon. "I feel like I can discuss almost anything with them now that they're adults."

"Even with your surgery," I added. "I haven't kept much from them. And I'm glad I haven't."

I glanced at Keith to see if he was in agreement.

"They've both been such good listeners," I continued. "I don't know what I'd do without them."

"Yeah, I know they've been good for you," Keith said, hesitating slightly. "And I know you need to talk to them. But sometimes I think you tell them *too* much, Gin. Especially about what's happening between me and you…some of the problems I've been having."

"Oh, Keith! I don't tell them *everything!*" I said with a sly smile. "But it's true, I do tell them a lot."

I curled my arm around Keith's. "It's not like they don't know about these things, you know. They're adults now, and they can appreciate some of what we're going through. Besides, they can tell when things aren't right between us—and then they worry."

We sat companionably for a while, watching the last ribbons of red-orange light turn to purple in the night sky. Sunsets were a favorite time of day for us, and we didn't want to spoil the end of this one with conversation.

When the light had faded to blue and grey, I spoke again.

"The issues we're dealing with are scary, hon: cancer, death, impotence. Steven knows he's at greater risk now because of your cancer. And what if this happened to him or Carew and we'd never shared anything with them about how we felt or what we did? I think it's *good* for them to see us dealing with our problems, instead of just trying to ignore them."

"Yeah, I know," Keith responded thoughtfully. "I understand it's important to keep them informed—and I *definitely* know they can handle it! But still...." Keith looked away.

He watched a chickadee struggle to loosen a twig from a pile of winter debris, finally breaking it free and flying off. Keith followed its erratic flight across the driveway and into the tall cottonwood tree.

He continued, sounding weary, "....It's not that I don't want the kids to know, Gin. It's just that it's a part of my life I'm very sensitive about. I feel like a weakling or a cripple right now, and I don't want the kids to pity me because I can't perform like a man."

I turned and looked Keith straight in the eyes.

"Don't *say* that about yourself! You're not a weakling or a cripple! You're just not completely *well* yet. You're still healing. It's only a matter of time until everything comes back," I said, trying to sound sure of myself. "We just have to be more patient, that's all."

"Maybe...but what if it never comes back? You'd think by now..."

Keith rose from the swing, picked a dead leaf off one of my newly potted geraniums and crushed it in his hand. He walked to the edge of the porch and let the pieces fall to the ground. I watched him standing at the railing, his head bowed and his shoulders slumped.

Then, suddenly, as if a cloud had passed over him and blown away, Keith lifted his head and straightened his shoulders, returning to where I sat on the swing. He flashed me a smile.

I loved his ability to shake off a mood like that, and I was glad to see him shed his dourness.

"You're right," he said in a much lighter tone. "I'm probably just being too anxious."

I moved slightly to make room for Keith.

"It's not in my nature to be patient, you know?" he murmured, reaching his hand up underneath my t-shirt.

Keith began nibbling my neck. "Maybe I'm not getting enough therapy."

I lifted my head to expose more of my neck. "Well then, I guess I better get back to my nursing."

Suggestively, I leaned into him

Keith took my hand and, with a lustful look, pulled me up off the swing. "Sounds good to me," he grinned.

As we headed up the stairs to our bedroom, I could hear Keith's voice behind me. "It's really all right to tell the kids whatever you want, Gin…Just don't tell *anyone else*, okay?"

Keith reached up and tickled my ribs.

I squirmed happily, then turned at the top of the landing to face him.

"Oh Keith, of course I wouldn't tell anyone else," I said, laughing and grabbing his hands. "But you *must* stop abusing your nurse, or you're going to be sorry…"

I quickly released his hands and tickled Keith back. Then, with a sharp turn, I raced up the hall, knowing Keith was close behind—anxious to share in the joy that was to follow.

For the short month of May and part of June our love life was a happy one. We enjoyed oral sex. It was fun, exciting and erotic doing "sixty nine," a position that had been an occasional part of spicing up our sexual repertoire in the past.

But by the end of June, the change in our situation was dramatic. After almost two months of exclusive oral sex, the novelty of orgasm without intercourse had become boring.

Even more of a concern was the fact that Keith's recovery was at a standstill. He still had not had the least sign of an erection, and we were discouraged and frustrated. With each passing day, the possibility of a return to our former sex life seemed unlikely, perhaps even improbable.

Our enthusiasm for lovemaking waned.

Laptop Notes, June 12, 1995

I never thought I'd ever get tired of oral sex. It was something I always dreamed of... having as much as I wanted. Turns out, ANYTHING can get old.

I'm tired of having sex like this. In fact, I'm getting tired of trying to have sex altogether. It isn't as exciting as it should be. I don't have the same feeling. I'm struggling to have an orgasm no matter what Gin does. It's like my desire is gone.

To top it off, my penis is shorter than before—like, <u>major</u> shrinkage! I know I've lost at least an inch or more. Those damn surgeons ruined me!

I'll never be the same again.

Journal Entry, June 15, 1995

I wish there was something we could do besides sixty-nine.

Oral sex has always been my least favorite way of making love. There's so much about it I don't like. I don't like having no eye contact. Feeling so separated.

The good part about sixty-nine is that we do have orgasms together again. And it's a little easier for me now that Keith doesn't get a hard-on or ejaculate...at least I don't have to strain to get my mouth over his penis, or worry about him coming in my mouth. But those things hardly make up for the rest of it.

I want to make love like we used to. To have Keith on top of me...or me on him. To look at each other. To kiss while we make love. To be held.

Oral sex was okay when we did it for variety, but doing it all the time is really the pits.

It was obvious to both of us that we needed to do something to expand our options, but we couldn't think of any way to make love other than what we were currently doing. Our frustration with the present—and our fear of the future—blocked us from seeing alternatives.

We were in a monotonous sexual holding pattern, and we felt trapped.

One night, Keith and I decided it might be a good idea to look for hints on how to rekindle our love life. Our hope was to find books written by couples who had gone through a similar experience, to get some practical ideas on what others had tried that "got them through."

I eagerly volunteered to check out our local Barnes and Noble as soon as possible, and cleared my afternoon calendar the very next day for a trip to the mall.

When I entered the bright, well-stocked bookstore, I headed directly to the aisle entitled "Sexual Pleasure and Performance." It was a large department, and took up an entire section.

Before I turned into the aisle, I casually looked around to ensure that no one was noticing where I was going. But everyone seemed preoccupied with their own searching or reading and paid no attention to me.

As I walked slowly down the row of shelves overflowing with books, I scanned the stacks for titles I might recognize. There were a few I had heard of: *Venus and Mars in the Bedroom, Growing Older Together.*

Then I noticed *Kama Sutra: The Art of Love*. This was a book Keith had often talked about wanting to buy. I reached for the large volume, turning aside so no one could see what I had chosen. I began leafing quickly through the pages. The photos were graphic, and aroused me—making me blush.

I quickly rechecked the area, making sure it was still clear. Then I turned back to the book.

Despite feeling uneasy over the possibility of someone —anyone—seeing me with the *Kama Sutra*, I couldn't put it down. I found myself looking longingly at the couples in the pictures. How I envied them. I wanted Keith and me to be able to do what they were doing. I wanted to try some of those positions.

It's so ironic, I thought. Just when I'm at a point in my life where I might have enough courage to buy such a book and put it to use, I can't. Bringing this into our home right now would be a slap in the face to Keith.

The book now felt heavy in my hands, and I put it back on the shelf. Maybe sometime in the future, I mentally sighed.

I turned back to scanning the stacks. Everything was written by psychologists, physicians, marriage counselors or sex therapists—nothing by couples.

I picked up a book with a subtitle that guaranteed "your sex life will improve after reading this handbook." I scanned the index. Aha! A chapter on impotence. Finding an easychair in an out-of-the-way corner, I eagerly began to read.

Impotence was defined as a temporary, treatable condition—something that could be corrected with time and patience. The author suggested techniques partners could use to help maintain erections, obtain stronger longer-lasting erections, or achieve erections. Techniques were outlined: oral teasing; manual massage with oils, creams, and food; and different positions.

The author proposed that one of the primary causes of impotence was due to "performance anxiety." A suggested cure for this was that couples refocus their attention from having intercourse to giving and receiving pleasure, in the manner of just touching and being touched.

I was encouraged by what I read until I came to the last sentence of the chapter. These words alarmed me.

"For impotence that is physical in nature, such as that caused by abdominal surgery, injury, certain medical conditions such as diabetes, or resulting from medications, *consult your physician.*"

I hurriedly pulled six more books off the racks. Quickly I skimmed the impotence chapters. I was dismayed at the similarity. Each author gave almost identical suggestions, and every chapter ended with the same disclaimer: "If your impotence is physical in nature, see your doctor."

That night, I summarized for Keith what I had learned. I skipped the part about impotence caused by surgery and illness, however, not wanting to discourage him.

"So where does this leave us, Gin?" Keith asked when I finished my book reports. "We've tried just about everything you read, and nothing's worked. Seems to me, your trip was a waste."

"I know, I know. That's what I thought at first, too," I agreed. "But we haven't tried this 'refocusing' suggestion. Maybe that'll do the trick. Maybe we've just been putting too much pressure on ourselves—or rather on you—and what we really need to do is back off for a while. Quit thinking about intercourse all the time and concentrate more on mood. We've kind of neglected that, you know."

Keith shrugged his shoulders in resignation. "I guess it's worth a try."

For the next few weeks, Keith and I touched, massaged and caressed. We lit candles, played music and read romantic poetry. We bathed together, rubbed scented oil on one another and danced.

The experience was wonderfully sensual, and reminded us of how important ambiance and touch are for "getting in the mood"—something we had been inclined to neglect in the course of our past "everyday" lovemaking.

We did our best to concentrate only on the moment, to become one with the music and think only of our partner's touch.

But we couldn't sustain our concentration for long. After a couple of purely sensual experiences, we digressed from touching for the sake of touching, to touching for the purpose of seeing if we could create an erection.

We were once again focused on intercourse. And frustration and failure immediately followed.

Laptop Notes, June 24, 1995

This touching stuff isn't working. It feels good and it's relaxing, but I can't keep my mind on it. When Gin touches me, I keep thinking about how her touch always used to turn me on and now, nothing.

It's demoralizing.

I just want to be left alone, but Gin keeps hounding me. Either she wants to talk about it all the time or "try again." She's really ticking me off.

She thinks I'm going to get over this, but I know better. This is how things are going to be. And trying to make love doesn't do anything other than remind me of the fact that my dick doesn't work! Hell, I already know that!

I just want to be left alone.

Journal Entry, June 28, 1995

The "touching only" thing didn't last very long. Now we're back to oral sex again.

I initiate lovemaking, thinking it will make Keith feel better, but instead it seems to make things worse.

Worst of all, in the middle of our lovemaking, Keith now asks "Is anything happening? Is it hard yet?" God, I hate when he asks that! I always have to say the same thing: "No. Nothing's happening." Then things really fall apart. Either he blows up and wants to quit right away or he gets silent and just lays there. In any case, he ruins everything. Of course he doesn't have an orgasm, and then neither do I.

There are times when I think maybe Keith is right. Maybe he really is impotent. But how would we know that for sure? He's certainly not trying very hard to get better.

He just wants to ignore the situation altogether. And maybe that's the way to go. I know I can't keep trying by myself.

"Well, Gin, let me tell you where our life could be headed," Keith said one night after a Prostate Cancer Support meeting.

His voice startled me. I had been sitting on our back deck, and hadn't heard the car pull up the drive.

"I didn't expect you home so soon," I said, tearing my attention from yet another beautiful, sun-painted Western sky.

"Yeah, well obviously, I *am* home," he replied, agitated. He pulled open a lawn chair and sat it down next to mine, the metal grating on the cobblestone patio.

"I want to tell you about the meeting," he said, never even glancing at the glowing streaks of light.

"Tonight, I decided to find out if any of the guys in the meeting were steered wrong by their doctors like I was, or whether I was the only limp-dick in the bunch."

Keith's cynical tone drew my full attention, and I turned my chair slightly so I could look directly at him. His jaw was clenched and his eyes were unblinking.

"So, shortly after the meeting began I asked right out if anyone in the room was having problems sexually. The room went dead. Everyone just kind of sat there and looked down in their laps. But then one of the older guys broke the ice."

"'OK,' he says, 'I'll admit it. I haven't been able to have sex since my surgery—but it's not a problem. In fact, I'm glad that part of my life is behind me. It's just one less thing to worry about.'"

Keith paused, and readjusted his chair with another noisy scrape.

"Then the group got *really* quiet," Keith continued, "'til the only other young guy in the group besides myself spoke up. And *he* says: 'Well, I'm having problems too. But I'm not about to give up. I'm doing everything I can to get it back... but it's a bitch.'"

Keith cleared his throat. "This guy says, 'I've tried all sorts of things. And right now my wife and I *do* have sex. But I can't believe how it's ended up. The only thing I can do now is what I used to think was 'kinky'.""

Again Keith paused. "And when that guy said that, I knew he was talking about trying to figure out how to make sixty-nine feel like the real thing. And I thought 'Yeah, that's right where Gin and I are. Either we have oral sex or no sex, there's no other choice.'"

The crickets were now the only ones making noise in the nearly dark night.

I spoke up, weakly—half-asking, half-pleading.

"Keith, there's *got* to be something else."

He looked at me, expressionless. "I don't know what else it *could* be, Gin. Without a hard-on, I'm pretty limited."

With that, Keith rose tiredly and went into the house.

I looked back to where the sun had been just a few minutes before, feeling bad. I knew Keith was unhappy with himself, with me, with his job, with everything. But what could I do?

I had tried everything I could think of and nothing had worked. I had run out of ideas.

As June ended, it was evident that Keith and I had lost the motivation to keep our sex life going. It had become too difficult to keep trying, when every time we made love we were disappointed.

It was unlike Keith and me to give up. We had always thought of ourselves as fighters, with a fierce determination never to admit defeat. But now, we just couldn't find the energy to continue. So we retreated. For the first time in our marriage, we used silence and avoidance as a way of evading conflict.

We took the path of least resistance. We stopped having sex altogether—and never said a word about it.

Looking Back
Disclosing our secret

Keith, on telling others...

My transition from desiring total secrecy in those early months to full disclosure today has been a progressive journey.

When I first felt that a return to sexual function wasn't happening, I, like most men who suffer from erectile dysfunction, was ashamed, confused and frightened. Impotence was difficult for me to discuss, and I certainly didn't want anyone to know about my problem.

But when Gin looked for help at the bookstore—hoping to discover wisdom for us through the experiences of others— she found nothing. And it was then that I began to realize how damaging silence can be.

Because no one else was willing to talk about their problems, we felt isolated—and at times questioned whether we were the only ones having trouble coping with this complex issue. But we knew this was impossible. Others, surely, were hurting just as much.

It was compassion that began to weaken my resolve to remain anonymous. In the second year after my surgery, Gin and I first discussed the possibility of us sharing our story. At that time, however, I insisted that if we did so, we had to use pseudonyms.

As time moved on and our relationship continued to improve, my confidence strengthened. I began phoning men from work who were newly diagnosed with prostate cancer, offering my support and assistance. The gratitude of these men was humbling, and further increased my belief in the need for a book about impotence, coping and "what *real* people do."

By the fourth year after my surgery, my commitment to reach out to others was total, and any need I had for anonymity had become unimportant.

I firmly believe people need as much information as possible on this subject. They need to know others have been through this and their relationship with their partner doesn't have to be compromised. They need to hear good sex is still possible.

If our book helps even one person get through this easier, I'll feel like we've made a difference.

Gin, on telling others...

In contrast with Keith's hesitancy to talk to others, *I* spoke with other people right from the beginning. Despite the fact that Keith asked me many times back then "not to tell anyone" about what was happening to him, I confided in the kids, my sister Karen, my sister-in-law Sue, and my good friends, Diane and Jean.

I told these individuals about our situation, because I, like many women, needed to "talk my troubles out loud." I was not seeking advice (at least not the kind I sought from a self-help book), but understanding and empathy. Good listeners that these people are, they provided that for me.

When I finally told Keith of my discussions with these people, we were well into the healing stage of our recovery. Consequently, he was at a point where he could accept what I did —acknowledging that I, too, had been hurting. Nevertheless, he still said he felt "somewhat betrayed and embarrassed". I've explained to him that my behavior was never intended to be disrespectful, but was rather, driven by a strong need to attend to my own mental well-being.

Today, Keith is grateful that I did what I did. He understands that releasing that tension helped me to persevere. He also realizes that, at that time—when I really needed to be listened to—he himself was too wounded to be able to hear me.

CHAPTER SIX

"I'm Gonna Give Myself A Shot in the Penis???"

"I'm going to have to call Dr. Barrett," Keith told me one morning in mid-July as we were getting dressed. "I'm having problems going to the bathroom. My stream is weak— real weak. And I'm having trouble getting it started."

I looked up from the edge of the bed, where I was putting on my stockings.

"How long has this been going on?" I asked.

"I noticed it a couple of weeks ago. I just didn't say anything about it."

Not saying anything had become the norm for us.

For weeks we'd been skirting issues, sanitizing conversations and avoiding spending time together. It was as if the discord that had crept into our sex life had now seeped into our relationship, contaminating the whole marriage. Since it was almost impossible for us to get through a day without a disagreement, we were, for the most part, silent.

"Well, you better call Dr. Barrett today and get this taken care of," I replied, making my way out of the bedroom.

Keith's voice trailed after me. "I'll do it this morning, from home, so there's no possibility of anyone overhearing anything…"

After breakfast, Keith placed his call while I cleaned up the kitchen. He spoke with Dr. Barrett for five minutes or so, and, while I didn't hear all of the conversation, I heard enough to notice that Keith's concern over his symptoms lessened as Dr. Barrett apparently assured him nothing was seriously wrong.

Toward the end of the conversation, however, Keith's voice sounded particularly dejected.

"Yeah, well, that part of me isn't working right either," he told the voice at the other end of the phone. "There's nothing happening."

When he spoke again, Keith's tone was a lot more positive. What, I wondered, had perked his mood?
Keith said goodbye, hung up the phone and leaned against the doorjamb. He looked pleased—even happy.

"So what did he say? " I asked, puzzled.

"He said it's probably nothing serious—just a stricture, a narrowing of the urethra. Pretty common after a prostectomy, apparently. He says it can easily be taken care of in the office."

Keith smiled. "But he said something else that was *really* interesting…"

Striding into the center of the kitchen, Keith stopped and stood straight as a soldier at attention before announcing: "He's going to give me the injections!"

The injections? For a moment I couldn't make the connection between the injections and the stricture.

Then it came to me. The penile injections! The injections Dr. Barrett told us about before Keith's surgery! The injections that would give Keith an erection "just like normal!"

"You're kidding!" I exclaimed. "He's going to give us the injections, so soon? We can have *sex* again?!"

"Yup," said Keith, smugly.

In an instant, my mind's eye raced backward and forward. Flashes of Keith and me making love, just like we used to, flickered through my brain. The pain of the past months simply melted from me, and I felt light and airy.

Life was going to be like it was before! Everything was now, truly, going to all right with us again.

I set the dish I was drying onto the counter with a clatter, and raced into Keith's arms. He caught me in mid-air, lifting me high off the floor and swinging me in circles. I held on tight, squealing with joy.

After three revolutions, Keith released me, both of us slightly dizzy. I turned from him, and marched around the room with my fists raised high, chanting: "Yes! Yes! Yes!"

While I skipped like a schoolgirl, Keith watched me and nodded his approval, a Cheshire-cat grin on his face. I grabbed his hand, bowed slightly and beckoned him to join me, which he did without hesitation. Our spirits soared as we danced around the sun-speckled breakfast room.

Finally our dance slowed, and as our energy waned we melted into each other's arms.

Keith gave me a strong, deep kiss. "I've missed you," he said, holding my face in his hands.

"I've missed you too," I replied.

Laptop Notes, July 15, 1995

I can't believe I'm actually going to give myself a shot in the penis! It sounds terrible, and it's got to be painful.

But I'm going to do it, no matter how painful it is. This waiting has been for shit. And I can handle anything for a couple of weeks, just to get things working again.

The shots <u>have</u> to do the trick. Because if they don't, what's left? I become a eunuch. Just what I thought would happen if I had this surgery.

So I'll give them a try, at least for a while.

God, it's going to feel good to have sex again!

Journal Entry, July 16, 1995
Thank God for Keith's stricture!!! Because of that little
stricture we're going to get the shots! We're going to be normal!
No more oral sex. No more fights. No more frustration.
Things are going to be good again. YAY!
I was really scared. Things were getting bad between us.
We weren't talking, we were avoiding each other, and we had
even stopped making love. We'd never done that before, and I
don't know where it would have ended up. After you quit making
love temporarily, how long does it take until you slide into
quitting permanently? Would we have gotten to the point where
we would never have made love again, ever? That's certainly
where we seemed to be headed.
I remember, months ago, saying to Keith that I wouldn't
miss making love to him. But I didn't expect it to be this way...
with us not even touching.
Oh God, thank you for rescuing us.

The day after Keith's call to Dr. Barrett, I eagerly told
Beth our news.

"...and then he said he would give your Dad the
injections..." I began, and proceeded to give her every detail of
what would happen during Keith's appointment.

"...then once he learns how to do the injections himself,
we'll be able to have real sex again!"

I concluded with a laugh: "I'm so happy I can hardly
stand it!"

"Great news, Mom!" Beth said, her enthusiasm nearly
matching my own. "It's been a long time for you and Dad!"

"I was thinking about something as you were talking,"
she mused. "You said that when they do that first test shot, you
two have to wait around the clinic for a few hours so they can
test its effectiveness, right? Well, why don't you and Dad have
your *own* test? I mean, why waste a good thing? Instead of

waiting around the clinic after the injection, why not check into a motel and enjoy it?"

That's Beth for you, I thought. Always ready to go just a step further than most folks.

I was so glad she and I were having a fun conversation. During the past couple of months, our phone calls had been depressing—mostly because of me. Whenever we talked, I had nothing pleasant to say. I complained about Keith, fretted about our future and, recently, vented my frustrations over our "non-existent" sex life. But now, thank goodness, that was behind us and things were looking brighter.

"Well, I have to admit, it's not something I'd thought about," I told Beth, smiling into the phone. "I'll talk it over with your Dad and see what he thinks."

At first, Beth's suggestion sounded way too risqué to me. Leave the clinic and go to a motel? What if something went wrong? What would we say to Dr. Barrett? And what would the people at the motel think when we checked in without luggage? I would be too embarrassed to do such a thing.

Still, I thought, it would be nice to go to a motel...

That night, when I told Keith about the idea, he immediately thought it was brilliant.

"That Beth," he said, beaming with pride, "she's my daughter, all right! Thinks just like I do! It's a great idea. Of course we'll do it!"

The treatment for the removal of the stricture was uneventful and painless, and when the procedure was completed, Keith got his injection. I waited nervously in the waiting area until a nurse came to tell me I could "join Mr. Laken now."

She escorted me to the exam room.

There was only one area for patient seating in the compact room, comprising a long built-in, upholstered bench, connected at one end to a small dressing room and at the other end to the doctor's desk. Keith was sitting on the bench, and looked up, cheerily, when the door opened.

The nurse stood near the door while I took my place next to Keith.

"The doctor will be in shortly," she said, closing the door behind her.

Instantly, I turned to Keith.

"So how did it go?" I blurted out.

"Great! Feel for yourself!" he crowed, looking down at his crotch.

I followed Keith's gaze to what appeared to be a bulge in his pants. I tentatively put my hand on the area that seemed the most promising, praying I would be able to feel *something, anything.*

"Oh my gosh, you're huge!" I exclaimed, pulling my hand back quickly, as if I'd touched a hot poker.

Keith beamed with pride. He took my hand, placed it back on top of the bulge and gently squeezed his palm over mine. Yes, there was no doubt—the shot had worked!

"Oh, Keith..." I moaned as I leaned over to him, being careful not to move my hand.

I gave him a peck. A kiss. A nibble.

Just at that moment, the door opened. In his typical fast-paced manner, Dr. Barrett was in the middle of the room within two steps. He glanced our way, paused for a micro-second, and then continued on to his desk.

Dr. Barrett busied himself shuffling papers, kindly giving us time to disentangle and readjust. Then we sat like stone pillars.

"So, now. Let me tell you how the shots work."

For the next few minutes, Dr. Barrett explained the mechanics of the injections, described the physiology of the penis and drew diagrams to help us understand just how the injections did their job.

I kept my eyes riveted on him, afraid to look at Keith or even steal a glance toward his crotch, for fear of breaking out in laughter. Like children in church who know they'll be unable to stop if they start laughing, I knew we both were willing ourselves to remain sober. I heard nothing of Dr. Barrett's words until he mentioned "leaving."

"...so I'll just give you this card now," he concluded. "It states that you should return in two hours to be rechecked. To help the time pass, why don't you two go have a nice lunch?"

Keith cleared his throat. "We're not really very hungry. We had a big breakfast."

"Well...okay then...Maybe you could do some shopping?" Dr. Barrett offered.

Keith stammered. "Well, um...actually, um...we thought, maybe..."

He took a deep breath, and when he spoke again, Keith's voice was steady and confident. "Actually, we were thinking of checking into a hotel for a few hours. To try this thing out."

Dr. Barrett looked up, surprised.

Then he smiled.

"Well all right then!" he said, with renewed energy. "Here's what I'll do. I'll leave the time on this card to read 'open,' and you two can take as long as you like in returning. Just be back here before five o'clock."

Dr. Barrett handed the card to Keith and started toward the door.

As he reached for the handle, he stopped and turned around. He returned to his seat, sat down, and rolled the chair into the middle of the room. Putting his hands on his knees, he leaned forward.

"I just have to tell you something," he said, grinning like one of Santa's elves who had just delivered a terrific Christmas present. "Being able to help folks like you makes me feel good. It makes me love my job."

He smiled broadly. "So, go do just what you planned. And have a *great* time!"

Before we left the clinic, we stopped by the pharmacy to fill our prescription for the injection and needles. Dr. Barrett had asked us to do this so Keith would be prepared for his teaching session upon our return. When the pharmacist discovered we were "first timers," he gave us a brochure about the use of the injections, and strongly urged us to read it.

"It has some good information in it," he noted.

I read aloud from the pamphlet on our way to the hotel we had chosen. It described the procedure of injecting, and had pictures and diagrams. The process really didn't sound too difficult. Keith would inject himself on alternating sides of the penis where there was spongy-like tissue; he would use a small-gauge needle and, if it was done properly, there should be no pain. We learned we could use the injections every three days, and the effects would occur within minutes.

Nothing seemed like too much of a concern until I got to one paragraph, which contained a sentence of warning. In heavy bold type, the sentence said, in part: "...if an erection lasts longer than three hours, seek immediate medical attention, as permanent damage to the penis can result from such a condition."

Keith looked at me quizzically. "Did you say a *three-hour* erection?"

On our way into town that morning, we had picked out the hotel we wanted to use for our tryst. It was brand new, and only a short five-minute drive from the clinic.

When we entered the lobby, we were struck by the fresh clean smell of new construction. The lobby was empty, which was not surprising in the middle of the day. Keith approached the desk while I hung back, trying to look nonchalant as I checked out the brochures in the tourist rack.

I watched from the corner of my eye as Keith checked in, and then quickly joined him when he was finished. On our ride upstairs in the elevator, we snickered like two teenagers playing hooky.

The large room had the same wonderful smell of newly hewn wood, and was tastefully decorated in mauve and a light shade of turquoise. We barely noticed the furnishings, however. Our eyes were only on each other.

Without speaking, we hurriedly undressed.

When Keith removed his shorts, I smiled lecherously at the size and rigidity of his penis. He walked toward me, and together we crawled under the fresh, clean sheets.

We touched each other hungrily, aching to explore and be explored, and we quickly moved to satisfy the urgency within us.

The intensity of our lovemaking was beyond anything we had ever experienced.

For the first time in almost six months I felt whole again. Complete.

We lay together quietly for a long time. There was no need for words. Eventually, we drifted off to sleep.

I awoke only when Keith stirred. "What's the problem, hon?" I asked dreamily.

"I don't know. I'm having some pain. I've got to get up and walk around."

When Keith released himself from my embrace, his penis was as hard and engorged as when we started our lovemaking—perhaps more so. We were both shocked.

I looked at the clock on the bedside table. The time had flown! It was now well over three hours since we had left the clinic, and Keith still had an erection!

"Keith, look at the time!" I shouted. "Remember what that pamphlet said? We've got to get back to the clinic to get you some help!"

We hastily tugged our clothes on. I drew a brush through my hair, Keith adjusted his pants and we hurtled out the door of our room.

In the lobby, we skidded out of the elevator, then forced ourselves to slow down, so we wouldn't draw attention with our breathless arrival.

We gave the desk clerk our key. It was the same young woman who had checked us in three hours earlier, and she avoided our eyes as she processed the bill and asked for Keith's signature. I could feel the color rise in my cheeks.

Once outside the lobby, we scampered to the car, revved the engine louder than intended, and sped off.

Arriving at the urology floor of the clinic, we approached the admitting desk with dread. Behind the counter was a nurse we had seen before: a large, intimidating woman who stood her post with the demeanor of Attila the Hun. How were we *ever* going to see Dr. Barrett without having to explain to The Inquisitor what was going on?

Keith held out his return card.

"There's no time on this card," she said brusquely, palming the card.

"I know," Keith replied, trying to swallow a hint of a grin. "Dr. Barrett said whenever I returned I could see him—right away."

The nurse gave Keith a hard, suspicious glance and told us, curtly, to take a seat.

As we waited in the lobby, I looked around. There were at least thirty other men waiting to see their doctors. Most of the them were older than Keith, and most were accompanied by women, whom I assumed to be their wives. They were all sitting quietly.

Keith however, was struggling to stay in his chair. He fidgeted, squirmed and crossed and uncrossed his legs—trying desperately to relieve his pain.

To our great relief, Keith's name was called within just a few minutes. He gingerly got out of his chair and moved toward the examining room. He looked awkward. His knees were slightly bent, and he walked as if he were trying to carry an egg between them.

Within ten minutes I looked up, surprised to see Dr. Barrett heading in my direction. He sat down next to me.

"Keith is fine," he began. "We gave him an injection to counteract the medication, and he's already feeling better. We'll have to adjust his dose and give him less next time. But we've decided that, given all he's been through today, we *won't* give him the instructions on using the injections himself. We'll put that off 'til next week."

Dr. Barrett patted my hand. "He'll be out in a few minutes."

Then he smiled broadly for the second time that day.
"Oh, and I got the results of Keith's PSA. Good news! It's still less than detectable."

In all of the excitement of the day, I had totally forgotten that Dr. Barrett had run a blood test of Keith's PSA level.

"Oh, I'm so relieved—about everything!" Instinctively, I leaned over and gave the physician a big hug.

Instinctively, he accepted it.

On the way home, Keith and I talked gaily about our day. Despite the little scare, it had really been a wonderful time. Keith's PSA remained undetectable, we'd had a *great* time making love, and our speedy evacuation from the hotel was a real riot in hindsight!

We laughed over the young hotel clerk who'd tried so hard to avoid looking at us; the irritation of the straight-faced, sergeant-like nurse, so annoyed with our unorthodox card; and Keith's fruitless attempt to hide his protruding erection from the other men in the waiting room.

Oh the embarrassment of it all!

But we were happy. We now had the "love potion," and everything was going to be fine.

Journal Entry, July 19, 1995

It's amazing to me how easily Keith and I have returned to conversation, laughter and fun again.

It feels so good to be in love and smiling. These injections are just what we needed. I actually feel married again! They'll carry us through until Keith is well.

Laptop Notes, July 19, 1995

I never had a clue a guy could have an erection so long it could hurt. But it did!

Next time I'll just use less.

Still, what a miracle. My ol' pecker was
really hard! The little captain rose to the
occasion, just like old times.
It was great!

The next week, Keith went out of town for a couple of
days on business. He returned home early in the evening on
Wednesday, and I met him at the back door with an amorous
kiss.

"Only two more days until you learn how to use the love
potion," I reminded him, squeezing his crotch. "Two more days
until we visit paradise again."

I twisted my head suggestively. Keith returned my
teasing with a deep tongue kiss, and fondled my breasts.

Over dinner, we told each other about our days apart.

Keith's meeting with his customer went well, and was
likely to result in a new account. I had presented a well-received
workshop to a new client.

I brought Keith up to date on the family. Duncan was so
upset when Beth had to take his blankie away to wash it, he just
stood in the laundry room and cried. Mom was still insisting she
could live alone, but had just had a bout with the flu that kept her
in bed for two days.

We talked easily, just like old times.

After dinner, Keith went to check his e-mail before the
10 o'clock news, so I waited in the family room for him to join
me. I lay down on the sofa and started to doze, but, within
minutes, was awakened by a movement in the room.

I looked up. Keith was naked, parading around the room
like a peacock.

When he turned to face me, I saw his large, engorged
penis.

My first thought was, "Keith is recovered!"

Then I thought again.

"Keith, what have you done?" I asked suspiciously.

"You like it?" he asked, ignoring my question and
swaggering closer.

"Have you given yourself a shot?" I accused.

"Yes I have! And we are going to have a *good* time!"

"But you haven't had the instructions yet!" I said, shaking my head.

"I read the book. It was easy. Look," Keith said, pointing to his erection, "I'm fine."

"But what about the dose? What if it doesn't go down?"

"Gin, don't worry," Keith urged. "I gave myself *half* of what Dr. Barrett gave me. Now come on. Don't spoil a good thing."

Keith sat down beside me and nuzzled my neck. "Let's just have fun."

I didn't need a lot of persuading, and I wasn't disappointed with my decision to give in. Once again, we had a great time making love.

Afterward, we were content and tired. We tried to sleep, but had little luck. Just as we seemed settled, one of us would pop up, lift up the covers and stare at Keith's penis. It was still as erect as when he first gave himself the injection. Then we'd drop the covers, roll over, and pretend to ignore what we saw—only to lay awake until the other person started all over again.

This process went on for nearly an hour before Keith got out of bed "to walk around a little."

"Are you in pain?" I asked worriedly, as he paced the bedroom, and then headed into the hall.

Keith didn't answer. When he came back into the room, he went straight toward the bathroom.

"I need some warm compresses," he said, taking a washcloth from the closet and holding it under the faucet.

Keith left again. I could hear his footsteps go down the stairs and into the family room. I knew he was going to sit in his favorite chair.

I got out of bed and dug around the bathroom drawer for the pamphlet about the injections. I read the warning, and looked at the clock. It was midnight now. Hmm. It was before the ten o'clock news when Keith gave himself a shot, I remembered.

I reread the warning. Rechecked the clock.

I repeated this routine two more times before I finally went downstairs. "Keith, it's been two hours now," I said with determination. "Let's call the clinic."

"No, I don't want to do that. I'll be all right."

Keith grimaced as he struggled to get up from his chair. "I just have to quit thinking about it and do something else."

For the next hour, Keith tried reading, watching TV and more compresses. Nothing helped.

At one o'clock in the morning, I couldn't stand it anymore. Pointing to the warning in the book I demanded, "We've got to do something, or you could really hurt yourself!"

Finally Keith gave in.

He placed a call to the clinic, and got an answering-service employee who took his number. Within minutes, a urologist called back.

The urologist told Keith that sometimes a decongestant, especially Sudafed, will work to counteract the medication. But he strongly recommended that Keith come to the emergency room in Rochester, because of the length of time that had now passed.

Keith got off the phone and rushed to the medicine cabinet. He frantically checked bottles, vials and packaged cold remedies. Finding no Sudafed, he downed four Contac and pulled on his pants.

"Okay, let's go," he yelled over his shoulder as he rushed past me, hurrying to the garage and buttoning his shirt at the same time.

The drive to Rochester was long and very silent.

Keith insisted on driving, despite his pain. I sat in the passenger's seat, vacillating between worry and frustration. (How I wanted to say, "I told you so!")

We arrived at the ER forty-five minutes later, just before 2:00 a.m. As we approached the admitting desk, I thought of how mortifying this situation had to be for Keith. How was he going to explain why he was here?

I was amazed when Keith confidently walked up to the desk and said, "I'm here because I have priapism." Somehow, he had remembered the medical term for prolonged erection!

The nurse escorted Keith to an exam room while I filled out paperwork and took my seat in the waiting area. Two other people sat quietly in the large chair-filled space. They were busy paging through magazines, and only looked up briefly when I, too, picked up a copy of the nearest outdated issue of something that, under normal circumstances, I would never actually considered reading—like *Motoring Through Canada On Your Harley* or *Redecorating In Red*. I flipped through it, seeing neither pictures nor articles.

I tried the newspaper. Halfway through the day-old sports section, Keith appeared.

"Let's go," he said, jingling his keys.

As we headed for the door, he whispered, "I'll tell you about it in the car."

When we were out of town and on the expressway, Keith started to talk.

"First of all," he said with a smile, "I'm fine." Then he chuckled. "But you're never going to believe what just happened."

I settled back, relaxed. Just by Keith's introduction, I knew I was going to hear a funny story. (And, at this point, Keith could have recited the phone book and I would have thought it was funny, I was so relieved he was all right.)

"First, this nurse takes me into an exam room and tells me I have to wait for another nurse to come in and get my history," Keith began.

"So I think, 'Okay, that's all right,' and sit down on a chair far away from the exam table. While I'm waiting, I'm thinking about my pain, you know—and wondering what's going to happen."

"Then in walks this beautiful babe. I mean *gorgeous*! She doesn't look like a nurse. She's young, with long black hair, and is wearing a form-fitting flight suit. And I'm like, 'Wow'. Then she reaches out her hand and introduces herself, but I don't even get her name, I'm just too mesmerized. She picks up a stool and moves it *right* next to me. She's sitting so close we're almost touching!"

"Then she says," and here Keith made a hilarious attempt to impersonate the nurse's sweet voice: "'I have to ask you some questions.'"

We both burst out laughing.

"She told me she doesn't normally meet patients," Keith switched to a tone of exaggerated seriousness. "Said her job is actually as a Medical Team nurse on the helicopter emergency flights, but, tonight, her unit was slow and she's helping out in the ER. The nurses had asked her to take this case because they thought it might be 'interesting to her'."

Keith paused briefly for effect. It was obvious he was having a good time entertaining me.

"Then she says, 'Now what exactly *is* your problem?'"

"You mean she didn't know why you were *there*?" I squealed.

"That's right! She didn't know *anything*—can you believe it? And when I told her I had priapism, she must have known what the term meant because she just says 'Ohhhhh,' very knowingly, as if she's just beginning to understand that she's been set up."

I groaned, then giggled. My response egged Keith on.

"But the worst is yet to come," he laughed.

"Once she's recovered from my diagnosis, she tries to be very professional again and starts asking me questions—boom, boom, boom. 'How long has your penis been erect?' 'Does it hurt?' 'Has this ever happened before?' 'Was there anything you did that might have caused this?'"

"I started to tell her about the surgery, getting the first injection, and giving myself half the dosage," Keith said, shaking his head. "But then she says, like she can't believe it, 'You couldn't wait to get the instructions?'"

Keith described how, at this point, he blushed and stumbled through trying to explain that he'd been away for a few days, hadn't had sex in a long time, and thought half the amount would be the right dosage.

"But she just stared blankly at me, as if she couldn't understand how I could do such a thing! Again, she says, 'You couldn't wait to get the instructions?'"

"Then," Keith chuckled, "like a miracle, I realize my erection's down and my pain is gone! I can't tell you how happy I was to be getting out of that room! I stood up and said, 'You know, I'm perfectly fine right now. I appreciate everything you've done, but I don't need any more medical help.'

"Then I tore out of that room without looking back!"

Tears were rolling down my cheeks, and my sides were aching with laughter.

"Oh Keith," I chortled, "I can't imagine what she's going to say in her report! Or the fun she's going to have telling the other women about this dirty old man who was so horny he couldn't wait to have sex—and then ended up with a four-hour erection!"

"Yeah, I bet she never thought a man my age would have this problem!" Keith smirked.

"All I could think about," he continued, "was how ironic this whole situation was. I mean, here I was, sitting next to this beautiful woman, sporting a hard-on bigger than *anything* I'd ever had, even as a teenager, and I can't even appreciate the moment 'cause I'm in so much pain."

I looked at Keith with mock sympathy.

"Well guess what, hon? It's not over yet. Tomorrow you have to tell this story again—when we keep our appointment with the urology technician who's supposed to give you *the instructions…* "

I shot Keith a stern look, emphasizing my words, "…on *just how to do* these injections!"

Keith looked at me, rubbed his fingers through his hair and groaned.

Then we both started laughing all over again.

* * *

Two days later, the children flew in to help celebrate Keith's fiftieth birthday. Everyone was in great spirits. We hadn't all been together in over a year, and the mood was festive.

Beth, Carew, Steven and Haley decorated the house with balloons and streamers. I got out the good china and made Keith's favorite dessert: carrot cake with lots of cream-cheese frosting. Duncan helped put the candles in place.

After a dinner of crab legs and beef tenderloin, we lit the cake and sang "Happy Birthday". We clapped and cheered as Keith blew out all fifty of his candles, a sure guarantee that his wishes would come true.

As we ate our cake, we started reminiscing. The kids asked me to tell some of our favorite family stories—the ones that always made us laugh no matter how many times we heard them.

"But I have a new story to add to our list!" I said, as I finished reciting the last of the vintage tales. "This is something that just happened the other night."

I glanced toward Keith, seeking his approval before I went any further.

He grinned sheepishly, laughed, and nodded his okay.

I eagerly leapt into my dialogue. I began with our appointment with Dr. Barrett, embellishing and dramatizing all the way. Within minutes, the kids were howling with laughter. Keith watched in delight.

As I got to the part about calling the Clinic, Keith stepped in to tell the rest of the story. He told about his frantic search for Sudafed, the voluptuous nurse, and his hasty escape.

When he was finished, we were all weak from laughter.

It was a wonderful party, and a beautiful weekend, together with our family—sharing love, laughter and our hopes for the future. What more could we want?

Keith was fifty years old. He had survived cancer. Our children were happy. We had a beautiful grandson. And our marriage was back on track.

All was well.

Looking Back
Finally, We Can Laugh

Humor and impotence from Gin's perspective...

Learning to appreciate the humor of our situation has followed a path similar to that of learning to talk about our experiences. It has been a journey with many twists—and one that often stops for a while before it starts up again.

During Keith's recovery, I vacillated many times over what I thought was funny. A situation that seemed humorous to me one day appeared tragically pathetic the next. And many days, I literally cried through my laughter.

Today, that confusion is gone. Now I can joke and tease right along with Keith about our "unconventional" love-making, and I can openly appreciate the humor of the moment. Like the time we forgot our vial of medication in an ice bucket in a California hotel, and laughingly decided it would be much less embarrassing to get a new prescription than to call and ask for it to be sent to us.

Having witnessed the healing that comes from laughter, I welcome it into our life, and often initiate it.

But timing is everything!

In the first year of our recovery, when Keith's emotional state could swing from high to low unexpectedly, it was difficult to predict how humor would be received. Consequently, I often misjudged Keith's mood or underestimated the stress of the moment, and any attempt at humor was received by Keith as being critical.

Thankfully, those times are behind us. As our relationship has improved, our sense of humor has fully returned, and now joking is once again an important part of our life.

I've discovered a similar evolution happens when we're talking with others who share our fate. When we swap stories, trust develops—and at some point we are able to move past the tears and share a good laugh together. And the beauty of that moment is wonderful—to laugh with others who really understand the bizarre and embarrassing nature of this problem!

Today, I'm not only *able* to do this, I want to do more of it.

Humor and impotence from Keith's perspective...

Before the surgery, I used to be right there with all the other guys, cracking jokes about guys who couldn't get it up, and making fun of short penises. In fact, I was probably the initiator of the jokes much of the time.

But not today.

Since my surgery, I don't crack impotence jokes or make fun of infirmities in public. I just can't. I'm too sensitized to the situation, and wouldn't want to hurt anybody who's trying to get his life back again.

But I *do* make jokes privately with Gin, all the time, about our *own* situation.

Why?

She and I have a unique sense of humor about this. We can now get a good laugh out of what could easily be seen by others as bizarre or tragic.

Some might call it "gallows humor," but I see it more as humor that's meant to relieve tension or to communicate feelings. Joking with Gin about my impotence helps me get things off my chest.

And I love double entendres, like "the little captain shouldn't go down before the ship" or "I can't keep a stiff upper lip."

Humor is strange that way. It's perfectly acceptable for me to make fun of *myself*, but no one wants to be the subject of jokes.

Like the old adage says: It's okay to laugh with me, but don't laugh at me.

CHAPTER SEVEN

"I Don't Want to Have Sex Anymore, Honey"

Laptop Notes, August 6, 1995
   These shots are amazing!
   I get a hard-on within minutes of injecting, and never have to worry about losing it. In fact, that's the only issue now—getting the dosage perfected.

Journal Entry, August 10, 1995
   This is wonderful...better than when we were first married! I can't get enough of Keith!
   We're using the shots every three days...and counting down the days in between.

Laptop Notes, August 21, 1995
   Gin is always telling me how good a lover I am and how much she missed me.
   God, I like hearing that. Makes me feel like a man again.

Journal Entry, August 23, 1995
I'll never take plain old wonderful intercourse for granted again. Never!
There's something so special about having Keith inside of me. It always makes me feel closer to him...like we're one.

Laptop Notes, September 7, 1995
Having trouble regulating the dosage.
First I get a four-hour erection that hurts
like hell. The next time I lower the amount and
only get half a hard-on.
Maybe I'll get lucky and we won't have to
use these shots much longer.

Journal Entry, September 10, 1995
Saturday we spent almost the entire day playing in bed, and when we finally got up, we never even got dressed!
It was great.

Laptop Notes, September 21, 1995
Making love every three days is beginning
to remind me of when we were trying to get
pregnant with Beth, and sex was like a duty I
had to perform. It became a job and wasn't fun
anymore.

Journal Entry, September 28, 1995
I'm having trouble knowing when Keith is "ready."
Once he gives himself the shot he gets an almost immediate erection...which in the old days meant he was turned on. But now it doesn't mean anything, other than he's given himself a shot.

But I shouldn't complain...not with what he has to go through just to even <u>have</u> sex.

Laptop Notes, October 2, 1995
     Every time we make love, I think "maybe this time." Then we start fooling around. And nothing.
     So I have to stop and give myself the shot. It puts me pretty much out of the mood.

Journal Entry, October 11, 1995
     The good part of Keith's not having an ejaculation is there's no dripping, but the bad part is I can't really tell when he has his orgasm. I miss the warmth of him inside me.
     It's just not the same.

Laptop Notes, October 13, 1995
     I'd give anything to have a quickie. To look at Gin, get a boner, lay her on the bed, and come without even thinking about it. I loved to start the day that way, with a quickie before work. Now, there's no way.
     Now I'd have to give myself a shot and have a hard-on for hours.

Journal Entry, October 21, 1995
     It's tough to keep my concentration when we make love these days. I'm always worried about what's going to happen when we're done. How long will Keith have priapism? Will Sudafed help the erection go down? Will we end up in the ER again?
     All the preparation and planning means I don't end up getting aroused. A lot of times I just fake it.

Laptop Notes, October 29, 1995
    Every time I try to have sex I'm reminded
of how mutilated I am. I've got scars on my
belly. I've got a penis that's an inch shorter
than before. And having to give myself the
needle just to get a hard-on is pathetic. How
can Gin even <u>think</u> about wanting me?

In only three months, we had gone from exhilaration
back to discouragement. No single incident clearly defined what
had happened, nor did any one moment identify the turning
point. Rather, a mixture of intertwined issues gradually eroded
our lovemaking and relationship.

These issues were diverse in nature, ranging from the
mechanics of learning to use the injections, and the resulting
changes in routine and spontaneity, to the persistent inability of
Keith to get an erection naturally.

Each of these factors affected our mood, self-image and
the way we related to each other. But no one issue weighed more
heavily than the continued absence of Keith's "normal"
functioning.

When we first began using the injections, we thought
they would be our temporary "love potion"—that all our
problems would soon be over. But now we were being forced to
see how naïvely optimistic we had been.

Weeks passed, and Keith's condition didn't change.
More and more, it become obvious that Keith was *not* going to
recover—that he was, indeed, impotent.

Accepting this painful reality was not something that
Keith and I did simultaneously. We each arrived at this point
separately, as the hope we were trying to maintain was slowly
chipped at by many small disappointments.

Not wanting to acknowledge the truth made us feel so
desperate that, at times, we acted in ways that were totally out of
character.

*   *   *

"I don't want to use the injections tonight," Keith said one evening as he followed me into our bedroom, taking off his polo shirt. "I want to give my old cock a chance to work on its own. Give it a test and see what it can do."

How casual and confident Keith sounded! Why, then, was I so hesitant? Nothing had happened in the last few weeks to give us any indication that Keith's penis could work by itself. Why was he looking for trouble?

"Hon, why not just lessen the amount and see what happens…you know…before we go cold turkey?"

I untied my sneakers and tried to sound as nonchalant as Keith had.

"No, I'd like to go natural tonight," Keith insisted. "I really think I can get it up."

Keith slid into bed and laid back on his propped up pillows, arms behind his head.

"And Gin, you know just what to do," he encouraged.

Troubled by Keith's expectations, I undressed slowly, then gingerly lifted the sheets and joined him. Keith drew me close, his hands rubbing up and down my back. His legs wrapped around mine.

I reached down to Keith's groin and began to massage. I used my hand, my mouth, my hand again. Despite my doubts, I prayed for a miracle. ("Keith deserves a break," I reminded God.)

But nothing.

"Why are you stopping?" Keith protested, when I quit stroking him and rolled onto my back. "Don't stop now!"

"Keith, my hand is tired! I need a rest. I've been at this a long time now."

I hesitated. "Maybe we should just give it up for tonight."

"Give it up?" Keith's voice rose in indignation. He put his arm around my waist and pulled me toward him. "I don't *want* to give it up! I want to stick it in you and drive you wild!"

"I appreciate the offer," I replied flippantly, "but I don't think it's going to work without the shots."

The word "shots" was barely out of my mouth before Keith was on top of me. Glaring into my face.

"I don't *need* the shots. I just need a little extra incentive," he growled. Then he reached down, grabbed his penis and started pushing his fist into me.

"Keith, what are you *doing*?" I asked in alarm.

"I'm going to stick it in! Then it'll get hard!"

Keith pushed again, trying to stuff his penis inside me. He pushed. He shoved. Over and over, he tried to make his soft organ go into me, but each time he failed.

Yet with each failure, Keith was more driven—more intent on succeeding.

He thrust again. Now his weight was becoming heavy on my chest, and his knuckles were digging painfully into my tender flesh, causing me to moan.

Keith pushed again.

I gasped.

Keith shoved harder.

"Stop! Stop!" I cried out, struggling to push him off my body. "You've got to stop! I can't take any more. It *hurts*!"

I felt rage, sorrow, and disbelief, all in the same instant. Who *was* this man? Not my Keith!

"I can't breathe! You can't just keep trying to shove it in when it isn't *hard!*"

Keith rolled to his side of the bed. I looked over at him. He looked confused and disoriented.

"What's happened to me?" he muttered under his breath.

For a few brief moments we lay there, dazed by the scene that had just occurred in our own bedroom.

Finally, Keith got out of bed and stalked to the window, slinging the covers to the floor behind him.

"Godammit! Just look what I've become," he stormed. "A eunuch. Good for nothing."

Inwardly, I sighed. Not this same old issue!

"Keith I know you're frustrated," I said quietly from under the comforter. "But it's not the end of the world. We've still got the shots."

Keith sat down suddenly on the bed with a thud. He lowered his head and shook it back and forth, as if trying to deny what he had just heard. He sat like this for a long while.

When he spoke again, Keith looked tired and beaten down.

"You're right Gin…you're right. We still have the shots."

Laptop Notes, October 25, 1995
Eight months after surgery and I can't get any kind of a hard-on. I know now I'm never going to get it back. It's over. Everything is gone.

Even my desire.

I've been stripped of that part of me that made me a man. I don't even care about sex anymore. If I never have it again, so what? I won't miss it, because I no longer even feel like it.

On the first day of November, winter arrived with a vengeance. An arctic front blew in from Canada, and within hours, the temperature dropped below freezing. The sky turned gray, foretelling a snowfall. As evening approached, gusts of sleet began blowing against the windows, each icy dart hitting sharply before sliding down the panes.

It was a Saturday, and we had spent the entire day catching up on household chores. I had concentrated on tasks that needed doing inside, while Keith winterized the outside of the house—draining faucets and mulching vulnerable plants. We had both worked hard throughout the day, but now, with our chores accomplished, we were relaxing in our favorite way:

sitting on the floor in front of the fire, coffee cups in hand, listening to Kenny G on the stereo.

"This music turns me on," I said breathily, as I put my cup on the hearth and nudged Keith's shoulder, trying to get him to put his arm around me.

"Yeah, I know."

Keith got up from the floor, picked a copy of a flying magazine off the coffee table and went to sit in his favorite chair.

Hmm, he's playing hard to get, I thought. He's been doing that a lot lately. Well, no matter. I can handle it.

I pulled off my sweater and started to crawl toward Keith, swishing my hips back and forth as I moved across the floor and lowering my chest to expose my cleavage.

I was certain Keith was watching me, even though he appeared to be reading.

When I got to his chair, I pushed the magazine into his lap, pressed my upper body on his and kissed him.

Although he accepted the kiss, he gave me none in return.

Undaunted, I sat back on my haunches and slowly began to take off my bra, exaggerating every movement. Looking directly into Keith's eyes, I flung the bra over my shoulder and asked coyly, "What's the matter, big boy? Too tired for a little fun?"

Keith dropped his head and looked down at the magazine.

"Hon, what's the matter?"

Silence.

"Keith, what *is* it?"

Keith looked up. His brow was furrowed, and his chin jutted forward. "Gin, I have to tell you something…"

The seriousness in his voice sent a shiver through my body. Keith looked down in his lap again, touched the magazine as if he was going to pick it up, then put it back down. He looked up, and swallowed hard.

"I've lost my desire to have sex, Gin. I've lost my drive, my libido. And I just…don't want to have sex anymore."

"You mean you don't want to have sex *tonight.*"

"No, I mean sex isn't something that's important to me anymore. It's not something I need to do…or want to do."

My heart started to pound hard against my chest, and I could feel my palms begin to sweat.

"Keith, I don't understand what you're saying. We have sex a lot. We just did it on Wednesday! What do you *mean* you don't want to have sex anymore?"

Keith put the magazine on the floor and leaned forward.

"Gin, I know we have sex a lot—like, almost every three days with the shots. But haven't you noticed that *you're* always the one who initiates it? I'm not *interested* in sex anymore. It's not something that's fun for me. I've only been doing it for your sake—going through the motions to make you happy."

My heart beat faster, and I felt weak. I wanted to get up off the floor, but the weight of Keith's words kept me from moving.

("…going through the motions…for your sake…it's not something that's fun for me…")

I glanced at the fire. It was beautiful—a glow of warm red embers. Cozy. Romantic.

("…going through the motions…")

The words chased each other around my head.

I looked up and became aware of Keith watching me. His stare made me feel ill at ease.

I realized that I was half-naked, and suddenly felt terribly embarrassed. I stood up, grabbed an afghan off the blanket rack and wrapped it around me. Then I moved to the sofa, where I sat in a tight bundle.

"Gin, I don't want you to feel bad. It's not about you or anything you've done. It's about me, and losing my prostate." Keith spoke quickly, like a child spilling forth with a long-overdue confession.

"I know they say losing your prostate doesn't affect your desire, but it *does.* When they took out my prostate, they took away my desire. And now, it feels like…sex means nothing to me."

Keith stopped. He looked around as if searching for something, then got up from his chair and went into the kitchen. I could hear him pouring coffee.

"You want a warm-up?" he called.

I couldn't answer. I was too busy trying to sort out what I'd just heard. If Keith had been going to lose his desire because of the surgery, it would have happened right away, wouldn't it? Not now! Keith had never mentioned this before, so where was he coming from?

Returning to the family room, Keith went back to his chair—far away from the sofa, and far away from me.

"Gin, are you all right? Say something. Tell me what you're thinking."

"Keith, I...I don't *know* what I'm thinking...or what to say."

"Let me try to explain it again," Keith said in a measured tone. "Before the operation, almost anything could make me to want to have sex. I could just look at you move a certain way, or see a picture of a pretty woman, or watch a sexy commercial on TV and I'd get interested. First I'd feel a sort of twinge in my groin, then that twinge would grow, and then I'd get an erection.

"But now," Keith continued resignedly, "I don't get that twinge. I look at you, a pretty woman, a sexy movie and... nothing. I don't feel anything."

My mind was whirling, and I felt icy cold, despite the afghan and the fire.

"Keith, I hear what you're saying," I struggled. "But it just doesn't make *sense* to me. Everything I've ever read about the prostate says all it does is produce the fluid that carries the sperm. It doesn't have anything to do with your libido."

"That might be what you've *read*," Keith answered, agitated. "But it's not true. I *know* I lost my libido when they took out my prostate! I know it, because *it's my body, and I know how I feel!"*

"My drive is gone," he stated flatly. "And nothing turns me on anymore."

I cringed, thinking how, just a few minutes earlier, I had tried to come on to him.

"So, you're telling me I'm not attractive to you anymore?" I asked, wounded. "Nothing about me turns you on?

For the first time that night, Keith looked at me tenderly. He got up to come sit near me on the sofa. But he didn't touch me.

"Gin, I'll always think you're a beautiful woman," Keith said consolingly. "And I'll always love you. But this isn't about being attractive or about love. It's about sex."

I couldn't look up to meet his searching eyes.

"I wish like hell that things *weren't* this way. I worry about how this is going to affect you," Keith said, seriously. "You're still young and healthy—you have desires and needs."

His fingers played with the fringe of the afghan.

"But I can't help how I feel. I can't keep making love when I don't have the drive."

My throat was dry, and my heart was beating so hard it felt like it was going to break through my chest. I wished I could turn back time. Start the evening all over again and do things differently. I'd give anything not to be sitting here, feeling so desperate.

But this was reality, and I had one more question I had to ask.

I took a deep, quivering breath and, looking up at Keith through tear-filled eyes, I whispered the question I was most afraid to ask:

"Don't you *ever* want to make love with me again?"

Keith reached over and took my hand in his, with a touch that was warm against my chilled skin. His expression was caring—and pained.

"Gin, I love you. And I'll be happy to help you out anytime you want. But for me…it's just not a need I have anymore."

Laptop Notes, November 2, 1995

I don't know what gave me the courage to tell Gin last night. It just seemed like the right time, and I had to get it off my chest.

I can't keep up the charade any longer.

What she's going to do about this, I don't know. She might get disgusted and just abandon me. Look for someone who can satisfy her.

No. She wouldn't do that.

But what <u>will</u> she do?

Journal Entry, November 2, 1995

I really can't believe what happened last night. Keith telling me he doesn't want to have sex anymore...that he's lost his desire. I couldn't believe my ears.

I know he's been upset about not getting an erection, but to say he doesn't have desire and doesn't want to make love. I just don't get that.

We can't just stop making love! We did that once, and it was awful.

I thought about this all last night, going over everything, and I'm convinced he didn't really mean what he said. He was just upset and frustrated because he can't get an erection.

I'm sure he's going through a phase, a natural stage of recovery. He's down right now and feeling sorry for himself. Heaven knows, he has the right!

But he'll get over this and be his old self again. I think the best thing I can do is keep coming onto him, so he sees I still want him.

This is no different from other times when Keith's been mad at me for something and said he wasn't interested in making love. But he never meant it then, and I don't think he means it now.

Keith has a huge sex drive. I can always get him interested if I really try.

I just have to be persistent.

For weeks I tried to implement my plan to entice Keith into making love. But I had very little success. My advances did little to interest him. In fact, they seemed to irritate him, and caused him to move even further away from me.

Contrary to what he had said, Keith rarely "helped me out." Most of the time, he either avoided me or rebuffed me. And during those occasions when he *did* give in to my requests, he made sure to remind me that he was doing it just for *my* sake.

The "phase" I thought Keith was in affected more than our lovemaking—it affected everything. Keith was now unhappy with almost every aspect of his life. He continually complained about his coworkers, lost his temper in meetings, and even hinted that he might look for another job. He avoided social occasions and didn't want to see our friends. He also had very few conversations with the children. When they called, he would quickly ask, "Do you want to talk to your mother?" and hand me the phone without waiting for an answer.

Impatient, and preoccupied with the worry that someone would "find out about him," Keith lost his wonderful sense of humor.

Now, his whole outlook on life seemed negative and angry.

One night after dinner, a couple of weeks after I had started my "plan," Keith got up from the table and told me he was going back to work.

"I won't be home until late," he added.

"That's fine," I replied. "I'm tired."

But I didn't mean it. I wasn't tired, and it wasn't fine.

I didn't want Keith to go. I wanted him to stay home and spend the night with me. But I didn't say anything because it really wouldn't have made much difference if he did stay home. He would still have avoided me, and I would still have felt alone.

I sat at the kitchen table for a long time that night. Sat and stared at the dirty dishes and the still-lit candles. I had tried to make the evening special: linen tablecloth, soft music, even his favorite meal—chicken au sage. What a waste it had all been.

I loved this man so much. He was my closest companion, my confidant. Keith was the man who had taught me to appreciate lovemaking, helped me overcome my hesitations and gave me such pleasure.

I missed my Keith, and I didn't dare wonder whether he would ever return.

Putting my head down on the table, I started to cry.

I can't give up, I thought. I have to hold on a little longer. Things will get better.

They can't get any worse.

Mom called us in the second week of November. She was having a lot of pain, and her doctors in Florida couldn't find the source. She was disgusted with their ineptitude, and, since she had always done her "major doctoring" at Mayo, she wanted to come to Minnesota and get a "good check-up."

"No problem, Mom," I reassured her. "Don't worry about a thing."

I tried to sound positive, but inside I was thinking: Here's *another* problem to deal with, when things are already so bad.

The oncologist was a compassionate soul. She held Mom's hand gently and spoke softly as she gave her the diagnosis. But nothing she could have said or done would have made the brutal words easier to hear.

"I'm so sorry. The cancer has spread throughout your abdomen. There's nothing more we can do. It's a matter of weeks. It's time to get in touch with Hospice."

That night, I was again the one who made the difficult calls: to Karen in Iowa, Rodger in Indiana, and my youngest brother, Harold, in Florida. I gave them the devastating news. Then, with a calm I didn't feel, I called Beth and Steven.

A week later, all of Mom's family—her children, grandchildren and great grandchildren, all twenty-six of us—gathered in our home to share Thanksgiving. The weekend was full of the joy of sharing memories, the sorrow of making plans and the inevitable pain of saying goodbye.

On Sunday, everyone left except Karen and Sue, who would stay and help Keith and me until the end.

All day Monday people kept delivering things: a hospital bed, a commode chair, a box filled with various plastic-coated sheets and pads, a bed pan, emesis basin and bedside table. By the end of the day, our living room was a disparate blend of welcoming salon and cold hospital room.

Our vigil had begun.

Within the first week, Karen, Sue, and I got into a routine. Karen would help bathe Mom and make sure she had all her medications; I would help her eat and do her hair; Sue would change the linens as needed and keep the room clean. We each took turns preparing meals, answering the never-ending phone calls and running errands.

Mom had only asked one thing of us, and that was not to be left alone. So we made sure that, regardless of our other tasks, there was someone with her twenty-four hours a day.

A devoted son-in-law, Keith shared in this loving duty with us. When he got home from work, he went right to Mom's bedside, told her about his day, did the crossword with her, and, on her bad days, silently held her hand. At night, all of us, including Keith, took turns sleeping on a cot by Mom's bedside.

These days were physically and emotionally draining. Each night, we went to bed exhausted, longing for refreshing sleep—awakening only to find it had often eluded us.

At the end of the second week, Sue got sick with bronchitis and was forced to return to Indiana. Quite unexpectedly, Karen's husband, Wally, showed up, telling us he "just had to come up and be there for Karen."

Journal Entry, December 10, 1995

I'm so jealous of how Wally treats Karen. He's really <u>there</u> for her—hugging her, kissing her, putting his arm around her, taking care of her.

I'm here all alone.

Sure, Keith helps out with Mom, holds her hand and cares for her. But what about me? What's he doing for me? I need him just as much as Mom does. I'm hurting too.

Keith gives me hugs and kisses only when I ask for them. And then they're not <u>real</u> hugs and kisses...there's no feeling in them. It's like he's afraid I'm going to want to make love or something, so he holds back. All I really want is for him to hold me. I <u>ache</u> for him to lie next to me and hold me.

Laptop Notes, December 12, 1995

I feel like I'm being pulled in so many different directions. Mom, Gin, work. Everyone wants a piece of me.

I just don't have the energy to deal with all of them.

I need time to sort things out. To figure out who I am and where I'm going.

But that's impossible. The house is always full of people, and every time I try to get away by myself, something needs to be done or Gin comes looking for me.

I appreciate everyone's help with Mom, but this is one hell of a rough time for me too.

During the fourth week, Mom's condition worsened dramatically. She was now totally bedridden, and her pain had increased substantially.

Our days became more hectic as we tried to keep up with the added care. Our nerves became frayed as we realized the end was drawing near.

* * *

"Keith, I need you to hug me."

"I *am* hugging you."

"No, I mean *really* hug me. Tight, like you mean it."

Keith pulled back from the lukewarm embrace. "Gin, I'm tired of you telling me what to do and how to do it."

I was tired too. Bone tired. The day had been especially trying. Mom had been restless all day and there had been little Karen or I could do to help her. We had tried repositioning, back rubs, increasing her medication—but nothing had helped her get comfortable.

Now it was almost nine o'clock, and Mom finally seemed to be resting.

But she looked so frail, so drawn, and her color was ashen. Karen offered to stay with her while I took a break. Concerned about Mom, I nevertheless gratefully took Karen up on her offer. Keith and I had been bickering off and on all day, and I wanted to settle things before we went to bed.

So now we were in our bedroom, where I was trying, unsuccessfully, to make up.

"Well, if I *don't* tell you what to do, you don't do *anything*," I snapped. "You never even *touch* me without me having to *ask* for it."

"Okay, okay, you tell me *exactly* how you want me to hug you, and I'll do it just like you say."

"Keith, this isn't about how you hug me," I said, exasperated. "It's about *wanting* to hug me. I want you to look at me and want me. To love me."

"Okay, okay. You want to make love. That's what you want me to do. Fine. But I'm not going to get the shots. We'll go 69." Keith grabbed my arm and started pushing me toward the bed.

"Right now. Let's do it."

"No, it's not *about* making love!" My voice shook with anguish as I wrestled away from his grip. "It's about *wanting* me,

105

holding me. Don't you understand that? Can't you be even a *little* sensitive and see what I need?"

"Sensitive? *Sensitive*? You think I'm not *sensitive*?" Keith was stung. "What about *you*? You're the one who doesn't understand what's happened to *me*. You don't realize that I'm not a man any more. That I always have to keep up my guard, to make sure no one knows what I've become. Especially from the people at work..."

"Keith, no one at work *cares* that you can't get a hard on!" I spat. "You're always so concerned about your job, your future. It's always about *you*. How about worrying about *us* for a change—about our marriage? How about worrying about *me*? Or about Mom?"

Keith's lips grew tight and white.

"Gin, don't you *dare* tell me I don't care about Mom! I *love* your mother. She's a great woman, and she was always a good wife to your Dad. She understood him."

The battle was fully engaged now, and the verbal barbs were intended to cause injury. They were hurled like well-programmed missiles targeted for the most sensitive sites.

And our aim was precise after twenty-eight years of marriage.

The engagement escalated rapidly as one of us resurfaced an old hurt and the other resurrected a forgotten promise. After twenty minutes, we were literally shouting over each other's words.

At the very height of the din, Keith threw up his hands and yelled at the top of his lungs: *"I surrender!"*

The abrupt silence that followed was almost as loud as the preceding battle. For a few long moments we stared at each other in silent astonishment as we realized the extent of the devastation we had inflicted.

Then Keith turned and marched out of the room.

I stood paralyzed. Despite the fact that every fiber of my being wanted to follow Keith, my mind would not let my body move. Karen and Wally were sitting with Mom near the foot of the stairs, and I couldn't bear the thought of facing them, even for a second.

Then I heard the sound of the garage door opening, followed by tires squealing.

I raced to the window and saw Keith's car peeling out of the driveway. In my mind, I could hear my own voice shouting: "Oh my God, he's left! He's gone!"

With my arms clasped around my chest, I paced back and forth in front of the dresser. A picture of us with Duncan watched me from the vanity tray. Our smiles were real then, I thought.

I stared out the window and replayed the fight over and over in my head. I went to the bedroom door, then back to the window for the second time. Where would he go?

Then my sister's voice broke into my thoughts.

"Gin? Gin? Gin...you better come down here."

Karen and Wally were sitting on one side of Mom's bed, holding hands. Karen's face was streaked with tears. Mom was asleep, but she looked grey.

"Gin, I think Mom's dying," Karen said in a ragged voice. "Her breathing's very shallow and it's..." She swallowed. "...irregular."

I collapsed in an empty chair on the other side of Mom. "She's dying? Now? Tonight? Oh my God..."

For three hours we sat beside Mom. We watched, waited and talked gently to her. We held her hand and wiped her brow. And we cried.

As I sat there, my emotions swirled madly, changing directions like the winds of a cyclone. I knew Mom and I had shared many good times together, but it wasn't enough. I couldn't believe she wouldn't be with me anymore. I didn't want to lose her! To never go on a trip with her again, to have to pick out fabric for a baby quilt alone, it just seemed too sad.

And where was Keith? Was he all right? I already regretted the hurtful words I had said to him.

One moment, I felt peace, knowing that Mom had enjoyed a really happy life. The next moment, my peaceful feelings were replaced by anger—anger that Keith had walked out on me and left me alone at this terrible time.

I was grateful I'd been able to have this time with Mom. Worried that my marriage was falling apart.

I prayed, trying to come to terms with all these thoughts. Please God, give me the strength to accept Mom's death. And please make Keith come home. I promise I won't be so mean to him again.

For three hours I sat there, my mind a seething mass of hurt and worry. I did my best to avoid Karen and Wally's glances, and was grateful they were making no mention of the bitter words I knew they must have overheard.

Then, the shock, the relief: Lights in the front yard! Keith was home!

Running to the back door, I threw it open and flung myself into Keith's arms.

"Keith, I'm so sorry, I'm so sorry." My lips pressed hard against his cold cheek.

Keith held me. Tight.

"I was so worried about you," I managed to utter, hugging him again.

Keith kissed me on the neck. A real kiss.

Then reality hit me. "Hon, we have to hurry. Mom's dying. Come on, before it's too late."

Keith was not too late.

Shortly after he took his place by Mom's side, she opened her eyes and asked for water. We stayed by her bed and talked with her until she started to doze off. Mom's color was better, and we knew the crisis had passed.

Leaving her in Wally's care, we returned to our bedroom. We said nothing as we undressed and prepared for bed. Only when we were in bed, lying in each other's arms, did we quietly say our apologies.

Then we, too, tried to sleep.

Journal Entry, December 18, 1995

Keith hasn't walked out on me since the first years of our marriage—early on, when we didn't know how to settle an argument. But that was twenty years ago! I never thought anything could ever make us regress to that point.

I've known for a long time we were in trouble, but I didn't think things were <u>this</u> bad.

Keith stormed out. I can't believe it happened. But it did.

What's going to happen to us?

Laptop Notes, December 17, 1995
    I'm ashamed of walking out last night,
but what else could I do?
    I was so mad, I just had to get away to
be by myself. Had to stop fighting with Gin and
think about things.
    My life is really disgusting.
    In my drinking days, I would have found a
bar and drowned my troubles, but now the best I
can do is walk the aisles of a 24-hour grocery
store.
    My life is pathetic.
    I know Gin is disappointed in me. I'm not
helping her. I'm not satisfying her. I'm
useless.

Exactly one week later, on Christmas Eve at 12:15 in the afternoon, Mom died.

CHAPTER EIGHT

Where Do We Go From Rock Bottom?
Advice From An Expert

The family room was warm and glowed with natural light, despite the fact that the temperature hovered near zero and the sun was more than an hour from rising. The light of a full moon streamed in the corner window, and the fading embers of last night's fire gave off enough heat to keep away the chill.

Dressed only in my nightgown, I still felt warm, cocooned on my couch, alone in the near-dawn solitude.

I'd been up for almost an hour now, awakened by a dream about Mom—a nightmare really. In it, I was so tired I couldn't get out of my chair to go to her bedside when she called me. Her weak voice had penetrated my deep sleep, calling over and over: "Gin? Gin?" But my body hadn't been able to respond. I couldn't wake up to go to her.

I'd awakened with tears in my eyes.

I had lain there in the dark for some time after waking, reassuring myself I had nothing to regret. I'd been attentive and loving during Mom's illness, and she had died peacefully, with me holding her hand and kissing her gently.

As my mind had eased, I'd thought I could go back to sleep. But other dark thoughts had begun to worm their way into my tired consciousness: cancer, impotence, a troubled marriage.

Sleep became impossible.

In the end, I had gotten up to try and untangle the knotted threads of my life. At this hour, for once, I had plenty of time to think.

"Gin?" Keith's voice was sluggish—and surprised. "Whatcha doing up so early? You all right?"

I was startled. Keith stood in the hallway, peering in at me, his eyes squinting. His tousled hair made him look young and boyish.

"Yeah, I'm all right. I just couldn't sleep."

Keith came and sat next to me on the couch, putting his arm around my shoulder. He looked at me with concern.

"I had a bad dream," I explained lamely. "And then I couldn't go back to sleep."

I rubbed my eyes with my fingertips.

"Another dream about Mom?"

"Uh huh. I dreamed… I was so tired of taking care of her that I couldn't move when she called for me. She kept calling and calling, and I couldn't get up."

I reassured myself aloud. "I *know* I did everything I could for her… It was just a bad dream."

Keith squeezed my shoulder.

I was grateful for his unexpected company. It seemed like a long time since we'd sat and talked—really talked. I'd done at lot of thinking during my early-morning reverie, and, now that he was here, I realized I wanted to share my thoughts with him.

"Keith, I need to tell you what I've been thinking about. Will you stay and listen?"

Keith looked a little apprehensive.

"Uh…sure Gin," he said hesitantly.

I took a deep breath and launched in.

"This dream helped me realize how tired I really am," I began. "Not just from caring for Mom, but from what's been happening to *us* too…I'm tired of fighting, and feeling lonely. I want it to end…"

Keith's face went pale. His brow wrinkled with worry.

I could feel tears prickle at the back of my eyes as I pushed on. "I want us to have a good marriage again."

Keith's eyes softened, and relief flooded his features.

"I've been sitting here tonight trying to figure out what's gone wrong between us," I told him. "And one thing that's come to me is that for months I've been living in a state of denial. Trying to pretend that everything about us, especially our sex life, was going to get back to what it was."

My throat was closing, and I spoke quickly to get all the words out.

"But tonight I finally let myself look at what's *really* happened. And the truth is, I know I can't go on pretending. I have to accept the fact that your impotence is permanent…"

I hesitated briefly.

"…because if I don't, we're going to stay stuck right where we are. And that scares me."

Tears started rolling down my cheeks. I reached for Keith's hand and closed my palms over his as if I were praying.

"Keith I'm afraid—afraid we might lose what we've worked so hard for."

Now Keith's eyes were filled up, too. He pulled his hand out from between mine and cupped my face. His voice was shaky.

"Gin, our marriage is the most important thing in my life, and I'd do anything to keep you happy, you know that…"

Oh thank God, I thought.

"…but that's what makes this whole thing so damn hard to live with. I want to be a good husband to you. But I don't how to do that anymore. Without desire, I have to *force* myself to get in the mood, which doesn't feel right. And then, there's the shots. Every time I use them, I'm reminded of what a failure I am. It makes me not want to keep trying. I can't face it."

Keith's depressed look made my heart ache, but I let him continue without interrupting.

"Gin, you use the word 'impotent' to describe me. And I guess that's the right word. But I shiver whenever I hear you say it."

His jaw muscles tightened. "I *hate* that word and everything it implies. Being '*impotent*' makes me feel like I'm just...taking up space. That I'm powerless to do anything for you —or anyone."

For the first time since our ordeal began, I didn't try to comfort Keith or persuade him that his perceptions were wrong. Instead, I listened to him quietly and intently.

And because I did so, I finally shared some of his pain.

"Oh Keith," I sighed, watching him blur through my tears, "we've both been so hurt...but we've turned away from one another. Why? Why have we found it so hard to comfort each other?"

The instant it was voiced, my anguished question pierced our hearts, and tore down our defenses. Pulled by longing and emptiness, we reached out to hold each other close.

And we cried, for all we had lost.

We sat, wrapped in each other's arms, until the sun came up that morning. The dawn of a new day seemed to give us the energy to look ahead.

Keith was the first to speak.

"Gin, I've been acting like a victim. Just giving up and letting impotence ruin my life. I don't want to keep doing that. I want to do something to help myself. The only question is *what.*"

He paused. "I don't know. Maybe I need to see Dr. Barrett again."

"Keith, listen...it's not just *you* who needs to change. I do too. We *both* need help. And somehow," I patted his chest with a fond hand, "we're going to find it."

Later that morning, I called Dr. Barrett, and brought him up to date.

"We're using the shots, but things still aren't good. Now Keith says he's lost his desire and doesn't even want to *have* sex anymore. We need some help Dr. Barrett, and…we don't know who to turn to."

The physician responded without hesitation.

"I think Keith's suffering from depression, Virginia. It's very common after someone has had cancer."

I could hear him scribbling a note. "I want Keith to see the chief of psychiatry here, Dr. Rome. If anyone can help, he can."

Dr. Barrett graciously offered to make the arrangements, and later that day his secretary confirmed that Keith had an appointment scheduled three weeks later.

Laptop Notes, January 10, 1996
    When I said I wanted help, I thought maybe Dr. Barrett would give me another kind of shot or something, not suggest a psychiatrist.
    That's one more thing to hide. Especially from Dad. All my life he's called shrinks "quacks" and said the people who see them are weak.
    Now I'm going to one.
    Well so what? Right now I'll use anything or anyone who might be able to help me.

Journal Entry, January 15, 1996

I'm surprised Dr. Barrett suggested a psychiatrist. I never would have thought Keith needed one—or that he'd ever agree to actually see one.

But once again he's surprised me.

In a way, his quiet acceptance makes me sad. It shows just how desperate he really must be.

During the time Keith and I waited for our appointment with Dr. Rome, our fighting eased dramatically. And our talking continued.

At first, our conversations felt awkward and stiff, and it was obvious we'd gotten out of the practice of really talking to each other. But in a few days, the ease returned, and, like good friends who easily pick up "right where they left off," we were soon able to share openly again.

During most of our time those three weeks, we talked about our losses, telling each other what we felt was missing from our relationship. We both felt unattractive—me, because my body no longer seemed to be enticing, and Keith, because of his scars and what he called his "mutilation."

I told Keith how tired I was of always being the one who had to initiate sex, and how I missed being wooed. Keith said he felt pressured when I came on to him so often, and that he needed more "breathing space."

While we came up with very few answers to our problems, we *did* do a lot of talking. At that moment in time, it felt like we *needed* to talk. And be listened to. Not once or twice, but over and over again.

Laptop Notes, January 25, 1996
        Finally, Gin's stopped telling me
everything's going to be okay.
        Not that I don't want things to be okay,
but the truth is, they're not.
        Now I can tell her how I really feel.

Journal Entry, February 1, 1996
        I feel like I've put down a heavy burden, and I'm focusing on where we go from here instead of always looking back.

        I don't know if we'll ever get back to a complete marriage again, but at least we seemed to have stopped going downhill...and we're talking.

As each day passed and the meeting with Dr. Rome drew near, we both grew nervous. Neither of us had ever been to a psychiatrist and we didn't know what to expect. What was he going to ask us? How personal was he going to get? Would he think we were okay?

As it turned out, our fears were groundless.

Dr. Rome was a gentle man, who, like Dr. Barrett, was around our age. His gracious manner and calm demeanor put us quickly at ease.

The session was an hour long, and would be divided into three parts, he told us. First, Dr. Rome would meet privately with Keith; then, since Keith was his patient, he asked Keith's permission to meet with me alone. Finally, the three of us would meet together.

During our individual meetings, Dr. Rome asked us to talk about cancer, death, healing, and recovery. He specifically wanted to hear our impressions of how Keith was doing, but did let us set our own agendas and talk about what was uppermost on our minds. Not surprisingly, Keith and I later learned that both of us had spent most of our individual time talking about the difficulties of dealing with our blighted sex life.

In the last part of our session, when the three of us met together, Dr. Rome gave us his impressions and recommendations.

"Keith, you exhibit some signs of depression, but nothing that's out of the ordinary for what you've been through," he noted. "Your depression isn't severe, and, personally, I don't feel you need to take any medication for it. In fact," he added encouragingly, "I think you're coping quite well with your cancer."

Keith and I both let out a long, loud sigh. Dr. Rome smiled broadly at our precision timing, nodding at our obvious relief.

"But I *am* concerned about how you're handling your impotence," Dr. Rome said plainly. "And I'm troubled by what you describe as your 'loss of libido.' I'd like to do some follow-up on this issue. First, I want to rule out any possible medical reason for your condition. We can do that by running some blood tests to check your hormone level. If we discover anything abnormal, I'd recommend you see an endocrinologist.

"But if we *don't* find any medical reason for your decreased sex drive," he continued, "I'd like to refer you to one of my colleagues, Dr. Don Williams. He's a specialist in the field of male sexual dysfunction and could certainly be of help."

We were speechless. Neither of us had heard of a specialist in male sexual dysfunction. This sounded exactly like someone we needed to see!

"Does this plan sound all right with you?"

"Sounds fine," Keith replied. "And...um...we could meet with Dr. Williams anytime. The sooner the better, in fact."

"Good. Stop by the lab on your way out for the blood draw, and I'll call you this afternoon with the results. If everything's normal, I'll have my secretary set up an appointment for you with Dr. Williams."

The blood work, indeed, turned up nothing, and we waited for a week to get a session with Dr. Williams.

It was a good week for us. We went to dinner at our favorite restaurant, talked about what we wanted to cover in our session, and snuggled close at night.

On the 45-minute drive to Rochester, our spirits were high; we were eager to meet "the Great Oz."

When we passed the hotel we had used the day we got the injections—the hotel we now called "our love nest"—we glanced knowingly at each other, smiling. We walked through the clinic holding hands, took the elevator up to the Counseling Floor, and waited anxiously to meet the man who would share with us the secrets to getting our sex life back in order.

At precisely two o'clock, the nurse called our name and escorted us to see Dr. Williams.

In yet another standard Mayo Clinic office sat a dark-haired young man, maybe in his mid-thirties. He stood up when we entered, and offered us each a firm, friendly handshake. He was self-assured, and projected an air of professionalism beyond his years. After spending a minimal amount of time in casual conversation, Dr. Williams suggested that we "get started."

Contrary to the private sessions we had had with Dr. Rome, Dr. Williams asked that we both remain in the room while the other partner spoke. We were asked individually to describe our marriage, and then to talk about the problems we were having.

As we each had a chance to tell our stories, the psychologist listened attentively, interrupting only to ask for clarification. He took lots of notes.

When we were both finished with our narratives, I asked the question we so badly wanted answered.

"Where do we go from here, doctor? I mean, what do we need to know to recover that…sexual closeness we used to have?"

Dr. Williams' response took us by surprise.

"You two are already well on your way to recovery— because you're talking to each other. The secret to recovery is to talk. Talk about all the things that are bothering you."

We leaned in, anxious to hear the next critical words. Surely he was going to tell us there was more to recovery than just *talking?*

"Becoming impotent causes a man to experience a tangle of emotions that can make him feel crippled and vulnerable. Before you can deal with these emotions, you have to sort them out. Identify them. Name them. Then you can take them one at a time and work through them."

"But the sorting process is critical," Dr. Williams emphasized. "That has to come first. The best way to do that, Keith, is by expressing your anxieties. And because impotence affects not just you, but your partner as well, this sorting must be done with Virginia."

"That's why I say you two are well on your way to recovery," he added, leaning back in his chair, "Because you're talking to each other."

Still holding hands, we squeezed each other's fingers.

"As simple as it may sound," Dr. Williams explained, "it's a major step that you two have realized the 'rules' of your lovemaking have changed—how often you want sex, the space you need. By accepting that fact, you've also accepted that you're going to have to create *new* ways of doing things that will be unique to the two of you. This isn't anything I can define or prescribe, or even anything that *you* can accurately predict right now."

"I would, however, encourage you to keep making love," he suggested. "Don't ever stop. Be experimental. Use anything and do everything you can think of that might help give you pleasure."

Keith and I glanced at each other and smiled sheepishly, each of us conjuring up graphic images. As we looked back toward Dr. Williams, Keith let go of my hand and shifted his weight.

"Dr. Williams, everything you've said sounds good. But right now, my biggest problem is that I've lost my desire. I don't have the *urge* to have sex anymore. And this is driving me crazy!"

Keith repositioned himself, tightly crossing his arms over his chest.

"If I'd known that the sex drive resides in the prostate, I'd never have agreed to that surgery. But no doctor told me that. They never said a *thing* about losing your drive when you lose your prostate. And now, I'm ruined for life!"

I watched him uncross his arms and curl his hands, making loose fists.

Dr. Williams turned his chair so he could face Keith directly. With genuine empathy, he acknowledged Keith's justification in feeling anger, frustration and resentment over what had happened to him. He talked for a few minutes about the feeling of being violated, and said he could appreciate Keith's distress.

Then Dr. Williams said he wanted to return to the issue of sexual desire and "drive," spending some time talking about the libido and how it works. He asked Keith if there were ever occasions when something caused him to think about having sex.

"Yes," Keith answered honestly. "If I see a pretty woman, a sexy movie, it can make me *think* of sex—but it doesn't make me *feel* anything, not physically anyway. My body just doesn't react like it used to. I don't get any kind of sensation to tell me I have interest."

Dr. Williams smiled ever so slightly.

"Keith, your reaction to seeing an attractive woman, your response of *thinking* about sex when you see her, and your interest in *looking* at her, all tell me you still have desire. Your libido is fine, and working quite normally."

I'm sure Keith was as puzzled as I was.

"Your problem isn't that you don't have an active libido," the psychologist offered, "it's that your *body's* been injured, and isn't working right. Desire begins in our brains—in response to things we see, smell, taste, remember. *They* trigger the brain to tell us we're interested. The brain then sends a signal to the rest of the body, telling it to respond. In a man's case, the natural response, of course, is penile erection and this is the sign most men take as telling them they have arousal. In your case Keith, this part of the sexual response—the physical response—has been damaged."

"And," he explained, "*that's* what missing for you—your ability to get an erection, not your libido."

Dr. Williams stopped and glanced out the window, allowing us to process this information.

"So…what can I do?" Keith asked after a few moments had passed.

"When a man is sexually dysfunctional from an injury like yours, he has to learn to do things differently," Dr. Williams advised. "He has to become more attentive to what his *brain* is saying versus what his *body* is saying."

"Consider this possibility for a moment." The psychologist held up a finger, gesturing toward Keith. "Perhaps what's happening in your case is that you're talking yourself *out of* arousal. I mean, you could be interpreting your non-erect penis to mean that you have no desire—when, in reality, you do, but aren't recognizing it."

The doctor leaned back in his chair, again. "If this is true, and I suspect it is, you're going to have to retrain yourself to become more intentional about acting on your initial instincts, no matter how slight they are. Trust that your body will follow and eventually respond—not with an erection, but with that urge you talked about."

Dr. Williams again let us sit with our thoughts for a short while before continuing. There was one more issue he said he wanted to cover: Keith's sense of feeling emasculated and incompetent.

When Dr. Williams brought up this topic, I thought for sure he was going to tell Keith he was overreacting (the feelings I had had about the situation for a long time). Instead, he did just the opposite.

Dr. Williams not only validated Keith's perceptions that a large part of a man's identity is entwined with his ability to perform, he also stated that it's "natural and normal" to feel inadequate when that is taken away. He told Keith it would take a lot of determination and hard work to regain his confidence and reframe his self-perception.

Then he turned to me. Dr. Williams said I could help Keith in this area. He encouraged me to listen to Keith *unconditionally*—to accept his feelings, withholding judgement, and be a sounding board for his venting when necessary.

"And don't take Keith's sexual rejections as anything personal," he cautioned. "Right now, Keith's rejecting you not because he doesn't love you or find you attractive, but because he's still trying to figure out how he feels about his own self image. He needs time to regain his confidence."

Dr. Williams ended our session by reminding us to be supportive of one other, to never stop making love, and, above all else, to keep talking.

Laptop Notes, March 1, 1996
        So I'm not crazy. Everything I've been feeling is normal AND my libido is okay. God, I needed to hear that!
        Of course women make me think about sex, but I never thought that was the same as libido. The brain/body connection is so intricate.

122

I'm just going to have to force myself to stay interested in sex, even when I don't think I want to.

If that's what it'll take to be horny again, then okay.

Journal Entry, March 5, 1996

It was so reassuring to hear Dr. Williams say the problems we've been having are normal. And nice to find out we're doing some things right!

We've been on such an emotional roller coaster...every time we thought we were okay, back we'd slide again. But now, maybe, we've found someone who can help us put it all together.

Why didn't someone tell us about Dr. Williams long before now???

Looking Back
Treating the Mind and Body

Keith, on treating the "whole person"...

The major turning point in my recovery from impotence occurred when Dr. Williams gave me that little bit of reassurance —that my suffering was normal, that we were on a good course, and that my libido was intact.

Nobody will ever know just how important it was for me to hear that.

Impotence is a prime example of the interconnectedness between mind and body. When a man loses his ability to get an erection, he loses more than a physical functioning, he also loses a part of his emotional and mental self-perception. To "fix" him, then, one logically must fix both the body *and* the mind.

Recently, I watched a PBS NOVA documentary entitled "The Truth About Impotence".

In it, Raymond Rosen, Ph.D., a psychologist at Robert Wood Johnson Medical School, made a statement that seems to support my belief.

"Sexual dysfunction does not occur in a vacuum," noted Rosen. "Sexual dysfunction is a dynamic dance, an interplay between two human beings. And the male's inability to get an erection may be a major stumbling block [in that dance]. It may be necessary or important to treat that and offer help for that particular problem; but we must always understand that this is only one small cog in the larger wheel of that couple's relationship."

In this same documentary, the producers of NOVA cite a well-known fact regarding the use of the injections: "....while the injections are effective in 80 to 90 percent of impotent men, nearly *half* of these men stop using the injections within a single year."

Today I totally understand the rationale for both of these statements.

While the injections gave me an erection, they did not *cure* me. I still had to come to grips with my perceptions of what being "impotent" meant. Like Webster's Dictionary, which first defines "impotent" as "weak, ineffective, powerless," I, too, defined myself as powerless. Consequently, I was embarrassed and hesitant to face Gin, even *with* the injections. Only until I got that part of my life "fixed" could I consider myself cured.

I'll never know what would have happened if Gin and I didn't get help from Dr. Williams. Perhaps I would have recovered regardless. But I highly doubt it. I believe I needed the help of a professional, and Gin has told me she felt *she* needed this help too.

Wrestling with the effects of impotence has been a mentally consuming experience for me. It has had a huge impact on my life, and, for a time, shattered my self-perception. Interestingly, if my arm or leg had been mutilated, I would have received help, as standard treatment, from a whole team of medical personnel—to fix my body, help me learn to function again *and* deal with my psychological trauma. I believe a similar approach should apply to the treatment of impotence.

Today, when I talk to others about erectile dysfunction, I'm not embarrassed to say that my mind needed help as much as my body. In fact, I readily advocate getting "total" treatment. I firmly believe that the mind-body connection cannot be ignored if one is to become cured.

And, frankly, I feel the medical community is remiss when they try to treat men otherwise.

CHAPTER NINE

Fumbling with the "New Rules" for Lovemaking

After our meeting with Dr. Williams, Keith and I felt more positive about our ability to recover our sex life. We'd already made some progress, apparently, and Dr. Williams said we had a lot going for us: good coping skills, a previously healthy marriage, and sound instincts. Buoyed by his assurances, self-confidence slowly returned in both of us.

We began to deal with our problems one at a time—as Dr. Williams had suggested—and started with the frequency of our lovemaking.

From the past year's experience, we had learned that regular and consistent sex was a vital component of our marriage. Without it our relationship suffered, and we felt distanced from each other. To keep our sex life active, we now knew we had to think differently about arousal. And since we couldn't rely on Keith's body to drive us into lovemaking, we had to become intentional about making sure it happened.

We decided that, for the time being, we would keep to a schedule. The every-three-days routine we'd tried when we first got the injections was too frequent, but I felt that the twice a month we'd had during December wasn't enough. We settled on at least once a week.

Keith asked me to watch the calendar and hold us to our commitment—and to be the initiator if necessary. He said that with his lack of physical cues he didn't feel up to the task, but said he *would* respond positively to my advances.

"I won't turn you away or avoid you, like I've done before, Gin," he promised. "I want you to keep at me. We *have to* keep making love."

From that day forward, we've made love regularly. The schedule, we felt, didn't "force us" into bed. In fact, it was an intense desire to get better that sparked our sex dates. We were eager to learn the "new rules" of our lovemaking. And the "sex schedule" and "no rejection" rules provided the security and safety we needed to continue trying.

Laptop Notes, April 3, 1996
     It seems awkward to start making love when I have no drive.
     I go though the motions, hoping my body will kick in, but it's hard to do things differently after all these years.
     Right now I'm using all my willpower to hang in there until something gets started. If I stay at it long enough, I <u>am</u> getting a stirring sensation. Not the way it used to be, but still.
     It feels like a weak memory of something trying to return.

Journal Entry, April 10, 1996
     It's clear to me that I have to be a much more assertive partner if Keith is going to get anything out of these "sex dates."
     It's not enough for me to just initiate sex and make sure it happens, I have to make it exciting. I have to do things to turn Keith on and keep him interested.

I think I was expecting too much of him before. I wanted him to walk when he was still crippled. Now I realize it's going to take a long time for us to figure everything out.

By the middle of spring, I started looking for ways to add variety to our lovemaking and to make the experience more exciting. I began to use candles, music, scented oils and lotions again, like I had so many months ago but had abandoned during subsequent months. I also "staged" our sex to occur in various locations—both inside and outside the house.

One evening I planned a tryst in our orchard, surprising Keith with a picnic and lovemaking under the apple trees. Another time I rented a room in a local hotel; we ordered room service, shared a jacuzzi and then made love.

I realized that, with the injections, we had fallen into a routine of making love only through intercourse, so I reintroduced oral sex, sixty-nine and mutual masturbation to add variety.

Being this assertive and sexually creative did not come naturally to me, and at times even embarrassed me slightly. But the fear of losing my marriage drove me to ignore my inhibitions and "do what had to be done."

In time, I began to feel more at ease, and even started enjoying the variety. And, as an added incentive, there was Keith's praise. He was pleased and humbled by my efforts.

"Gin, you totally amaze me," he said one night as we lay in each other's arms after trying out a new position. "I never thought you had it in you to come up with some of these ideas!"

I laughed and nestled closer to him.

"It means a lot that you're trying so hard to help us out. If I didn't have you," Keith sighed, "I think I'd have been too discouraged to keep trying. Things are moving so slowly, I'm sure I would have just given up by now."

We were making progress in small steps, and our recovery was going well. But we still experienced frequent and persistent setbacks.

There were many times when our lovemaking seemed to depress Keith more than excite him. The pain of priapism sometimes negated the pleasure of orgasm. Other times, the injections seemed to remind him too much of his loss, and then he wouldn't want to continue. And always, Keith struggled with discouragement over his lack of desire.

When his spirits were low, Keith's mood swings would vary drastically, as they had during the previous year and a half. At one moment he could be sad, the next resentful. During these periods he would often belittle himself, reverting to the name-calling he had done so often in the past: "worthless", "useless", "not a man."

Or he would start second-guessing his decision to have surgery, saying, "I should never have just accepted Dr. Barrett's biased opinion like I did. I should've looked at radiation more thoroughly. Talked to more people. Like guys who had surgery and did become impotent. They could've told me how things really are. Instead I just let myself be led to the slaughter..."

Often, Keith's mood shifts occurred after we made love. As we lay in the dream-like state of emotional letdown, Keith would become melancholy and start longing for his former self.

"Our sex is good, but I'll never feel like a real man again," he told me on more than one occasion. "I'll always miss that passion I used to feel. The feeling of getting a hard-on, the surge of coming..."

Usually, though, Keith would realize the uselessness of his despair, and would quietly recoup.

"I try not to think about these things," he whispered to me one night after a mournful conversation. "Because when I do...I just get too sad."

During these episodes, I tried hard to be the sounding board Dr. Williams had suggested. I was learning to listen to Keith's pain—waiting until he got it all out, and empathizing with his feelings.

Journal Entry, May 4, 1996

I feel so bad about all those months I spent discounting Keith's despair. How many times did he try to talk and I didn't listen? How could I have been so foolish?

For God's sake, I teach these communication skills, and it still took Dr. Williams to help me see how wrong I was.

I'm beginning to understand how deeply this issue cuts to the very heart of a man's psyche. I think I can now appreciate that it's natural for a man to feel impotent...when he's impotent.

At one point during the summer, Keith's frustrations ran so high that he had a blow up with a resident at the Clinic during a recheck of his PSA. The rechecks always made us nervous, reminding us of Keith's vulnerability, and for weeks before the appointment we were both tense and edgy.

"I hate this waiting. Why can't they *ever* be on time?" Keith grumbled as he stuffed a magazine back into the rack, tearing the back pages.

It had been a long day at the Clinic. Keith had his blood drawn at 8:00 a.m., and we had waited until 2:00 p.m. to get the results.

"Did I tell you I talked to Beth yesterday?" I asked, trying my best to ease the tension. "She's so excited about having this next baby at home. I told her we're *both* going to take time to be there to help with everything."

Keith brightened immediately.

"Yeah, how about that, Gin? Another grandchild! And November's a perfect time for me to get away from the office. End of the year's always slow for orders and sales calls."

Before Keith could get any further, the door opened and the doctor entered. He was a young resident, certainly no older than Steven, dressed in a tailored suit and crisp white shirt. He shook our hands and mumbled an introduction, avoiding eye contact. Then he went to the desk at the end of the room and busied himself leafing through Keith's chart.

For what seemed like at least five minutes, the resident flipped back and forth through pages of lab tests, doctors' notes, and surgical records. Finally he spoke, rattling off the results of Keith's recent test with the detachment of a man checking off a shopping list.

"Your PSA continues to be less than detectable. That's good.

"Not having problems with urination. Good.

"You've been using the injections for over nine months. Also good."

The young man kept his eyes focused on the papers in front on him.

"Everything about your chart looks good. So you must be quite pleased with how things have turned out."

Keith glanced at me, lifting his eyebrows and rolling his eyes. Then he spoke.

"Well actually I'm *not* very happy about the way things have turned out," he answered, in a tone deeper than usual.

For the first time, the resident looked up at Keith. He seemed perplexed.

"What do you mean?" he asked, with a challenging tone in his voice. "We've saved your life. What more could you want?"

"Well doc, how 'bout a sex life?" Keith returned snappishly. "That's what more I could want!"

The resident inhaled slowly.

"You don't seem to understand," he patronized. "You're probably *cured* of cancer. How can you complain about your sex life, when you're lucky to be alive?"

Keith looked the young man squarely in the eyes.

"What kind of life do I have?" he retorted, now speaking quietly. "There's something called 'quality of life', doctor. And, frankly, sometimes I don't think I have as much quality anymore."

Keith's voice gradually rose again as he spoke. "I just want to be normal. To enjoy sex with my wife anytime I want."

"But you have the injections..."

"Let me *tell* you about the injections," Keith interrupted curtly. "Have you ever really *thought* about them? Just how do you think it *feels* to have to stick a needle in your penis every time you want to make love?"

"But you're fifty years old," the resident began. "So sex...".

Since it was obvious that nothing good was going to result from this debate, I took the opportunity to interrupt.

"You know, how 'bout if we finish this discussion with Dr. Barrett?" I offered.

"I think that's an excellent idea," the resident concluded, slapping Keith's chart closed and heading toward the door.

Keith and I watched in silence until the door was completely shut.

"What a jerk," Keith said.

"Yeah, what a jerk."

Within a few minutes, Dr. Barrett entered the room.

"Good to see you again," he exclaimed, extending his hand to each of us. "You both look great!"

Dr. Barrett placed Keith's chart on the desk, and, in his usual style, pulled his chair close and leaned forward.

"So how are you doing, Keith?" he asked. "I hear from my resident you're having some problems."

For the next few minutes Keith unloaded on Dr. Barrett. He told him about his frustration with the shots, his concern that his desire was never going to return, and the anger and despondence he often felt.

As he talked, the agitation in Keith voice lessened. When he was done venting, he paused momentarily.

"But things *are* getting better," Keith concluded. "We've been to see Dr. Williams, as you know. And he was a big help. He told us some things we didn't know before. And lately, Gin and I have been trying a few new things...experimenting a little."

While Keith was speaking, Dr. Barrett listened, nodding his head occasionally, and waiting until Keith was completely finished.

"Keith, I know you've had a hard time, and I'm really sorry about that," he stated with feeling. "This is a rough situation. There's the cancer and the surgery, then pain, incontinence, impotence. It's a lot for a person to contend with."

He paused, only for a moment.

"But you *will* get through this. It may not seem that way right now, but you will. And, while it's hard for you to believe, someday you'll probably even be glad you had the surgery."

Keith looked down to the floor. He sat quietly for a moment before he spoke, still with his head down.

"I suppose you're right," he replied. "It's just that sometimes things begin to pile up, and it's hard to see past them. Then I get a guy like your resident there...and I just have to let loose."

The summer passed, and by the time fall arrived, Keith and I had accepted as "normal" the fact that, for us, lovemaking would forever begin as a mental rather than physical process.

There was little spontaneity in our sex life. No more waking up in the middle of the night for a spur-of-the-moment "sleeping pill." No more lunchtime rendezvous. Also, we couldn't rush things in the passionate, urgent way we sometimes had before. And not having Keith's strong desire to turn me on anymore now meant that, I, too, needed plenty of time and an ample supply of patience to get going.

Starting to make love unaroused meant learning to trust that the body would eventually follow the mind's lead.

For me, as a woman, this approach to sex wasn't really completely new. I had frequently been motivated to have sex when my body wasn't yet aroused, for the sheer pleasure of meeting my husband's passion. But for Keith, starting to have sex unaroused was a radical shift from normal.

During those first few months, Keith was very tentative about beginning to have sex when he had no urge to drive him and when he was doubtful of his capability to regain desire. But as the months passed and we continued to make love consistently —working together to give each other sexual pleasure— Keith realized that his body could indeed *develop* arousal. Given enough stimulation, he could again experience some of the lust he thought he had lost completely.

But even as Keith realized he *could* experience arousal, he now had difficulty *maintaining* his desire.

"It's so frustrating!" he would say. "Just when I think my body's really getting turned on, I lose it! My drive is weak. I just can't seem to hang onto it."

At first, Keith tried to increase the strength and longevity of his desire by going through the motions of being an assertive lover—thinking that perhaps his body could access some latent memory of his past strong libido. But that didn't help much.

Then he tried experimenting with the timing of the injections.

That made a big difference.

As soon as Keith changed from injecting himself *during* lovemaking to *prior* to lovemaking, his arousal and sustainability increased dramatically. Now, within a few minutes of foreplay, Keith's body "kicked in" and he experienced an urge that felt more natural to him than anything he'd experienced in the last two years. His desire responded to my touch, increasing and decreasing as we progressed through lovemaking.

"It's not as strong as before my surgery, but it's enough to keep me interested," Keith told me. "Knowing what it feels like to have *no* interest, I'll take this any day!"

Changing the timing of Keith's injections was a major breakthrough for us. It not only helped him get aroused and sustain the feeling, it also altered our attitudes toward *using* the injections.

Once again, just like when we first got them, we saw the injections as a vital component to our love life—a means of keeping lovemaking alive. And, for the first time, we could even see advantages to using them.

Laptop Notes, November 14,1996
    I feel like a teenager again!
    With this good dosage I figured out, I
can get an erection as hard as when I was 19.
Or better! And I can keep it up for <u>at least</u> an
hour with no pain.
    I'm not worried about losing it anymore,
or coming too soon and spoiling it. Now that I
can have sex without caving in, I can really
work on getting Gin turned on. And that makes
things even better.
    Maybe these shots aren't so bad after all.

    With Keith's new level of responsiveness, the intensity
of our lovemaking increased significantly, and we thought we
were now recovered. We assumed that things were as good as
they could get. Love had returned to our bed, and we were
content.
    But we had not arrived at the finish line of our recovery yet.
    As the year came to a close, we were about to experience
one of our most significant breakthroughs yet.

Looking Back
Libido and Arousal Are Two Different Things

Keith, on libido and arousal...

Little has changed since the early days of my recovery. My libido continues to function fine, but my arousal has never fully returned.

Thanks to Dr. Williams, I now see libido and arousal as two distinct but interrelated factors in the sexual formula.

When I speak of libido, I'm talking about the attraction or interest I have in sex—the "pretty-woman-makes-me-think-about-sex" reaction that Dr. Williams referred to. Arousal, on the other hand, is what I call the automatic response of my body to satisfy that interest. In this regard, I'm not the same as I was before my surgery.

In the past, if Gin would give me a sexy kiss in the morning, I would find myself getting more and more horny during the day—so much so that, by evening, I felt I *had* to have sex with her to satisfy my body's craving. But that's not how things work today.

These days, when Gin gives me that same kiss, I'll think about it during the day and then gladly make love with her that night—but not because of the pull of my body. Now I do so because I have sustained my interest by mentally anticipating the pleasure I will get and give.

I can't say, however, that I have no automatic arousal. If it has been a while since Gin and I have made love—like if one of us has been on a trip—I'll often get a weak "woody" during the night, or perhaps even during the day. But the drive is weak and I can't sustain it. Within a few minutes, the erection subsides, and I'm likely to be distracted by other things.

I think I'll always miss this part of my sexual response. I liked the feeling that my body was on fire and being driven to satisfaction. I still, however, consider myself lucky. I'm able to develop arousal during foreplay and can still experience great orgasms.

And, given that fact that I'm now 56 years old, I might have been in this exact place anyway, even without my prostatectomy.

Gin, on libido and arousal...

For a couple of years, the timing of what Keith called his "loss of desire" puzzled me. I was confused by the fact that if it was going to occur, why didn't it happen immediately after his prostatectomy?

But lately this inconsistency doesn't trouble me as much.

I've learned to accept the fact that, when it comes to impotence, or to any medical condition really, the exception is the rule. No two people will react in the same way to their condition. Nor is there any prescribed course to follow. Consequently, I now accept the timing of Keith's loss as "his" timing.

Additionally, I used to question what exactly happened to cause Keith's libido and arousal to diminish? After all, he wasn't on any medication or taking any treatment that might affect him, nor is he a diabetic. So what could it be? Then I thought about the times I've "lost" my libido—times when I didn't feel well, was sad, tired, or even too busy to think of sex. There was no logical explanation for my "loss" either.

So for the time being, I'm not worrying about the why anymore. Instead I'm content to just enjoy the moment and our times together, and letting the sexual mysteries remain mysterious.

CHAPTER TEN

Overcoming Impotence—A Second Time

"It's almost the New Year," Keith mused. "Hardly seems possible it's already here, huh?"

I nodded my head and glanced at him. Keith, like me, sat comfortably in a chaise lounge, stretched out on the balcony, as the sounds of the evening tide came in.

The breeze was soft and warm, and my lips tasted slightly of salt.

We were spending New Year's in South Carolina, at a wonderfully deserted resort right off the coast of Charleston. We had been there for four days already, and it had been just what was needed. We'd played golf every afternoon, walked the beaches two or three times a day, and ate fresh seafood at quaint restaurants.

Being away from home for the holidays had seemed like the right thing this year, on the first anniversary of Mom's death. We'd both needed a change of scenery and time alone together. But we had also been torn by wanting to be with family. To solve our dilemma, we'd spent Christmas with Steven and Haley, then left the following day for South Carolina to usher in the New Year.

"Yep, it's been quite a year. So much has happened." I took a sip of white wine, laid my head back and closed my eyes.

Keith reached across the few inches of space between us to take my hand.

"But it's been a good year, Gin. A really good year."

"I'm glad you think so, hon." And I was. "I agree."

We sat companionably for a while, thinking our own thoughts. Another dusk was upon us, and a light breeze ruffled my hair.

"So," I asked, turning my head, "what's been the most significant part of the year for you, hon?"

"That's easy," Keith answered. "There are a few: your Mom's death, Galen's birth…and the recovery of our sex life. Without a doubt."

"Not being cancer-free?"

"Yeah, of course, that too. I mean, two years of remission is wonderful. But I see that as part of what makes Mom's death and Galen's birth so important to me. Surviving cancer makes me see those things differently than I would have before."

Keith looked out at the darkening sky and inhaled the sea air.

"Being there to help your mom leave this world in peace —that was such a beautiful experience. And then, in the same year, to be there to see the birth of my grandchild. To watch this precious little being take his very first breath, and hold him when he was still wet."

Keith's eyes shone in the fading sunlight, and he gently squeezed my hand. "I just can't say how much that's affected me."

"The entering and the leaving, and I got to witness both of them this year. It was a gift—an honor really. I don't know why I got to do this, but it's made a difference in the way I think about life. How precious it is. Not something to be wasted or taken for granted."

He stopped and smiled. "I'll never forget it."

I returned the smile, feeling warm and happy.

"You're such a beautiful person," I told him, with love in my voice. "I'm so happy I'm married to you. And that you're still here with me."

For the next little while, we sat holding hands and listening to the rhythmic roll of the waves—like a heartbeat, bringing life and energy to the world.

Then we watched the stars fill the sky.

When the air became cool, we both decided we were hungry, and went in to the kitchen, to prepare the two large lobsters we'd bought for a celebratory New Year's Eve dinner.

After a delicious meal, we licked the butter off our fingers and decided to take a stroll on the beach under the light of a half-moon.

Walking the shoreline, we further reviewed the year's events: the pain of our fighting, the insights from Dr. Williams, the arduous journey of recovery. We each took a turn expressing a wish for the future. Keith wanted to eventually feel "normal" again. I wanted to continue to free myself from my inhibitions and be an adventuresome lover.

When we returned to our condominium, we went to bed to celebrate the New Year.

Our mood was light and happy, and we were relaxed in our lovemaking, knowing that the injections gave us plenty of time to play. We joked, teased, and had great fun arousing each other. Keith surprised me by producing a feather, which he lightly ran over my body, making me shiver in delight. His creativeness spurred me to suggest using some whipped cream we had in the fridge as an extra "taste treat". We lovingly toyed with each other—enticing, then backing off, then enticing again. When we did finally made love, the experience was vigorously delightful.

"That was great!" I breathed at last. I could feel an ear-to-ear grin splitting my face.

"Glad you enjoyed it, My Lady," Keith laughed, affecting a British accent. "My only wish is to please you."

"Well you certainly did that, Squire."

Keith looked down at his still-erect penis. "So why not enjoy yourself again?" he asked, with a wink and a lecherous grin.

I blushed from head to toe.

"Oh Keith, I couldn't," I said, suddenly timid.

"Why couldn't you? Go ahead," he urged. "Use me! I'd love it."

But I still held back.

"Oh hon, I don't think so."

I felt hesitant about acting in such a self-serving manner. But then I remembered my New Year's wish, and I thought again.

What am I afraid of? I asked myself. Just what do I think might happen if I tried something new? Who knows—I might like it. And if I *don't* do this, I might regret it some day. You never know what tomorrow may bring.

With those thoughts in mind, I knelt up, threw my leg over Keith's hips and did exactly as he had asked: I used him.

Not once. Or twice. But multiple times.

And it was wonderful!

Journal Entry, January 1, 1997

What a night last night was! I feel like I gave myself a precious gift: abandonment. For the first time <u>ever</u> I totally let myself go and gave myself permission to do <u>whatever</u> felt good. It was fantastic, both physically and mentally.

I feel free—released! Like I've finally taken the last step in ridding myself of my sexual hang-ups.

Last night, I experienced sex for the pure pleasure of making <u>my body</u> feel good. And the more I enjoyed myself, the more Keith urged me on. The whole thing was so sensual.

This was the first time I ever really accepted Keith's body as a gift to myself, purely for my own enjoyment. When I was done, amazingly, I felt no guilt about it.

Finally I let myself acknowledge my <u>own</u> cravings, and enjoyed sex for no other reason than to make <u>me</u> feel good. Hallelujah!!!

Laptop Notes, January 1, 1997

For years I've dreamed of having a woman want me so badly she couldn't get enough. Last night, that dream came true.

Gin just let herself go and jumped my bones. She climbed on top and used me over and over. It was awesome watching her get off on me!

I felt more like a man last night than I've felt in a long, long time.

By the summer of 1997, two and a half years after Keith's diagnosis, we seemed well on our way to recovery. We were enjoying lovemaking again, our marriage was strong, and our self-esteem was almost restored. We no longer felt rejected or unattractive anymore.

Our healing was primarily due to our continued commitment to practice what Dr. Williams had suggested: to be supportive, to never stop making love and to keep talking. By being mindful of these simple phrases, we had been able to rebuild and reestablish our sex life, not to what it was in the past, but to an even better, more intense level of pleasure and awareness than we had had before.

We were now more focused and intentional about making love, wanting each and every experience to be as interesting and exciting as possible. Overall, we had become more conscious of "attending to" both our sex life and our relationship.

It was clear that we needed to stay open to change, and always be willing to try new things. We now understood that, to ignite passion, we had to ignite interest. And because we were more in sync with each other, we once again started hugging, kissing and "playing" with each other—and *not* just when we were making love. Now, our "signals" were not just used as invitations to go to bed, but rather as indications of our mutual desire and commitment to keep our love life alive.

Because of the struggle to overcome impotence, we had a new appreciation for the vital role that physical intimacy plays in our marriage, and we vowed never to forget the importance of touch. During the months when we had avoided physical touch, we had both been starved for it, and the scars of that hunger were, in a way, permanent. Because of them, we would never again take for granted the ability to share our bodies. Like surviving cancer, overcoming impotence had made us more grateful for every day, more appreciative of our time together and more aware of the fragility of life.

After almost three years, Keith had, for the most part, stopped thinking of himself as useless, worthless and incompetent. As Dr. Williams predicted, this re-framing had taken a lot of determination, and was a long process, comprised of many steps. Success at work, the security of knowing I was working *with* him, our contract of having "sex dates," my increased desire for his body, and our improved communication were all factors that helped Keith restore his self-image. But then, there was also the incremental return of his ability to be aroused, appreciation from men with whom he shared his experience, and the respect and admiration of his children.

Ultimately, however, it was Keith's strong belief in "giving back" that allowed him to get past his self-deprecation. He didn't want to waste any more time either feeling sorry for himself or not living up to his potential.

Our progress—individually and as a couple—had been nothing short of remarkable, and we were pleased. We thought we had weathered the worst of our problems, and looked forward to the future, optimistic that things could only get better.

"Peyronie's Disease? What's that?"

With the portable phone in hand, Keith was striding around the kitchen like a caged tiger. He had placed a call to Dr. Barrett and, as I watched him pace, I felt his anxiety.

Last night, when we'd tried to make love, Keith had been in a lot of pain, because of a bend in his penis.

He had first noticed the bend, which really started out as a slight curve, two weeks earlier, and hadn't thought much of it. But then the curve had worsened. And making love had become almost impossible.

"You can fix it, can't you?" Keith's voice was strident. "There *is* some way to get rid of the bend?"

I held my breath, and watched Keith's stricken expression with dread.

"So there's no hope?"

Keith listened a short while before saying goodbye and hanging up the phone.

"Damn it!" he yelled, stomping toward the family room, but immediately swerving in the kitchen doorway. "Damn it!"

"What did he say?" I asked solemnly, putting a cup of coffee on the table at Keith's usual place, and sliding into my own chair.

Keith sat down and picked up the cup. But he didn't drink. He winced, and shook his head from side to side.

"Dr. Barrett says I have something called Peyronie's Disease. That's why I have the bend. It's caused by trauma to the penis...and there's nothing they can do to fix it."

Keith put the cup back on the table and fingered the handle. His voice cracked slightly.

"He says I might not be able to have intercourse anymore...that he's really sorry...hopes I won't give up..."

Pushing the cup away, Keith stood up and slammed his chair under the table. Again he walked in circles, talking.

But I had stopped listening. I'd heard enough.

I sank down deep into my chair and looked out the window. The swing on the large hickory tree caught my eye. Keith had put it up last season, in anticipation of our summer visit from the grandbabies, and now it hung empty, pushed around by the autumn wind. Empty, just like I felt.

"Gin! Are you listening to me?"

I looked up, jarred by the nearness of Keith's voice. He was sitting next to me again, rubbing his hands over his face and through his hair.

"Oh Keith," I wailed suddenly, my sadness welling up and boiling over. The tears were hot, and stung my eyes. "How can this be *happening* to us?"

I started to reach for Keith's hand, but only had enough energy to reach part way and let my hand lie limp on the table.

"What are we going to do?" I sobbed once more.

"I don't know, Gin. I don't know."

For the rest of that day and the next, we said very little to each other. We were despondent.

The news of Keith's Peyronie's had thrown us off balance, making us retreat into solitude. We avoided each other during those two days—not because we were angry, but because we needed time alone to figure out how to face this.

Laptop Notes, September 9, 1997
    I can't believe this shit!!!
    Peyronie's. Who ever heard of Peyronie's? A bend in your penis. Where do these things come from? And why did I have to get it? It really pisses me off!
    I could become impotent again.
    But I'll be damned if I'm going to go through that whole victim routine again! This time is going to be different.

Journal Entry, September 13, 1997
    These past two days have been awful. The sadness, the worry...it's just like before. I can't even stand to think about it.
    What if we lose everything?

We can't let that happen. We've got to keep working
together, holding on to each other, being there.
We can make it through this. I know we can.

On the morning of the third day following Dr. Barrett's
diagnosis, Keith and I talked about our feelings during our
morning walk. We told each other how we both wanted to fight
to work though this crisis, and needed to maintain some sense of
control over our destiny. We knew we couldn't just give up. We
had to do *something*. So, together, we devised a plan.

We decided that we were going to engage in intercourse
as often as possible, for two reasons. First, because if we weren't
going to be able to enjoy it for much longer, we never wanted to
look back and think we hadn't taken advantage of opportunities.
Second, we thought that the use of the injections and the pressure
of intercourse might actually lead to a cure.

Our hypothesis was simple. We rationalized that "forced
erections" and the friction of intercourse might "break through"
or at least stretch the scar tissue that had formed in Keith's penis
—enough to allow the surrounding connective tissue to expand
and to free the penis from its bend. Of course, our theory was
completely unproven—a layman's approach to medicine. And it
might not work. But we were eager and willing to try it out.

"After all, we've got nothing to lose," Keith rationalized.
"Why not go for it?"

For the next four weeks, Keith endured the pain of
getting an erection and performing intercourse with a penis that
didn't want to straighten, while all I could do was hold him and
watch him suffer through it. His determination was inspiring, and
his perseverance amazing.

"Keith, are you sure you want to keep going through
with this?" I asked one night, as he grimaced through sex.

"Gin, I'll do anything I have to," he replied through
gritted teeth. "Until there's no hope left."

Our lovemaking was more meaningful to us now than
ever before. Not only could each sexual experience be our last

opportunity to have intercourse, but every time we made love it seemed to me to be a symbol of the increased resilience of our marriage, a reminder of our capacity to survive *whatever* the future had in store.

For a month, we didn't know whether our plan was working, but we didn't give up. We kept to our schedule and performed intercourse, despite Keith's pain.

Then, in the sixth week of "working our plan," we noticed a slight lessening of the bend.

By the eighth week, there had been an even greater decrease.

By the third month, the curve was gone altogether.

We had won. We had *not* given in, or let despair overtake us. We had not allowed Keith to become impotent for a second time.

Journal Entry, December 10, 1998

No matter what happens in the future, I now know beyond a doubt that Keith and I can face it. We have the love— and the resolve—to conquer anything. We may not like what we have to face, but we can face it, and live through it.

That's a powerful thing to know.

Laptop Notes, December 15, 1998
I have no idea what the future holds. Something else could happen to make me impotent again, I suppose. My cancer could come back. I could get hit by a car and be paralyzed. I really don't know.

But what I do know is that right now I feel strong. I'm going to live every day to the fullest. I'm going to play with my grandkids, encourage my children and love my wife.

It can't get any better than that.

Looking Back
What We've Learned About Being Lovers

Gin, on experimentation...

When I let go of my inhibitions that New Year's Eve and experienced multiple orgasms from "using Keith," I thought I had reached the pinnacle of my sexual experimentation. But, in reality, I had only reached a small plateau.

Since that night, sexual exploration has become a part of my life. And I couldn't be more thankful!

I've finally learned that nothing is "wrong" or "bad" about sex—including devices, positions or toys—as long as Keith and I agree that we *both* want to use them. It's fun, interesting, and in many cases, necessary for us to use sexual variety to keep our physical intimacy alive and active.

And now I know I'm not alone in my thinking.

I monitor an on-line discussion group of people who are suffering from impotence due to prostate-cancer treatment, and I've been amazed and inspired by the lengths to which some people in this group will go to get their sex lives back. I've learned that when it comes to restoring potency, "anything that works" is a possibility, and should be considered without guilt or embarrassment.

While Keith and I don't do anything that could ever remotely be considered "bizarre," I am conscious of keeping an ever-open mind to possibilities. I'm willing to try new toys, read sex-improvement books, and challenge my own instincts to continually make our sex life as interesting as possible.

And not only am I having more fun and enjoyment in my relationship with Keith, but I realize I could have been doing this all along.

Keith, on being a lover...

Today, I feel I can satisfy Gin like I've never been able to before—not just because of the sustainability I have from the injections, but because I've learned how to be a more considerate and engaging lover.

Our sex now, while it *has* lost its spontaneity, has gained intensity. We have a sort of "meeting of the minds" as to when we're going to make love, and we block off time for it to happen. Days beforehand, we start hinting of what we have in mind. So the planning process itself actually intensifies our lovemaking.

Then there is the act itself. Because I no longer have to worry about "the puppy going down," I can concentrate on Gin more than I used to. And afterward I can extend the process to seconds, thirds and fourths for her—giving me the satisfaction of providing a level of sexual pleasure I didn't know I was capable of.

If I lost the ability to engage in intercourse, I think I could still be a great lover to Gin. I'd still be compassionate, caring, understanding, and physically giving in *any* way I could to make her feel good.

I've learned that there's no greater satisfaction in my life than for me to remain close and intimate with my wife.

CHAPTER ELEVEN

Our One-Night Stand with Viagra, the Little Blue Pill

It seemed like 1998 was going to be a memorable year for us.

In May, we would go to Baltimore to watch Steven and Haley present their doctoral dissertations, and receive their degrees from John Hopkins. This was something we'd all anticipated for the past five years. What an accomplishment! And how proud we would feel when the day actually arrived.

Then in August, we would again return to Baltimore, this time to hear Steven and Haley exchange their wedding vows. They had decided to have a small, personal affair, and had asked Keith and me to give a short talk during the ceremony, offering our thoughts on marriage. We were very honored.

Finally, the year would end with the birth of another grandbaby. Beth and Carew announced that a third child was due in the fall, and we couldn't be happier. They're wonderful parents, and we were pleased they were really having that large family they'd talked about.

We felt truly fortunate. Our hope had always been that our children would contribute to society, leaving the world a better place than they had found it. And they were exceeding our expectations.

Actually, there were many things that were now going well in our lives. Keith was feeling good, our relationship seemed to be healthy again, and our sex life was back on track after the short detour with Peyronie's disease.

The new year offered some interesting possibilities for our sex life, too. Just a few weeks earlier, the FDA had approved a new drug for the treatment of impotence: Viagra.

The preliminary media reports about Viagra seemed almost too good to be true. You could take the pill daily, up to two hours before engaging in sex, and develop an erection in response to sexual stimulation. The medication was reported to have a low incidence of side effects, and the pharmaceutical community was calling it the "cure for impotence."

Keith and I, like thousands of others, were anxious to try this miracle drug. From all we had read, Viagra offered some distinct advantages over the injections: We wouldn't be limited to the number of uses in a week, there were no reports of priapism, and using an oral medication alleviated one of the major concerns of long-term injection use—developing injection-site scar tissue.

Even with all of the possible benefits, however, we did not rush to Dr. Barrett's office as soon as Viagra was available. Instead, we waited for three months, until it was time for Keith's check-up.

I suppose our patience was due to the fact that we were content with how things were going for us. Since the Peyronie's scare, our lovemaking had continued to improve steadily, and had even increased in frequency and variety. We regularly enjoyed oral sex or "quickies" with the vibrator, or our very favorite: "gourmet sex" weekend dates, where we would spend an entire Saturday or Sunday in bed. Our sex life was now the passionate, exciting and satisfying experience we had long ago talked of—once the children were grown and we were "sexually free."

Still, we were curious about Viagra, and always looking for ways to make things even better. So when Keith's check-up was due, in May of 1998, we asked Dr. Barrett for the little blue pill.

"I'm not surprised by your request," Dr. Barrett said with a slight chuckle. "I think I've written more prescriptions for Viagra in the past two months than I have for any other medication in my entire career! And I've seen men come into my office who I haven't seen in years."

"Well, you know how it is with us horny old guys," Keith said easily. "We can't get enough!"

Even though Keith couldn't truly describe himself as "horny" these days, he still had his sense of humor. I sat back and laughed, pleased with how content my husband now seemed.

It was good to see Dr. Barrett again, too. He was so kind, and always ready to listen. During the past four years, our relationship with him had developed, and now he seemed like both a doctor and a friend.

Most of this appointment, in fact, had been spent catching up on each other's lives. Dr. Barrett was interested in Keith's new company, and also wanted to hear all about our grandchildren; he, too, was pleased to hear about the new one on the way. We, in turn, wanted to know how his career was progressing, and of any interesting discoveries he was working on.

Even in the Clinic setting, it was easier to be relaxed these days. In the past four years, Keith's PSA had never risen above "undetectable," and there was every reason to believe he had survived his prostate cancer.

"So you'll give me a prescription?" Keith asked.

"Sure, I'll give you a prescription." Dr. Barrett answered, "But I want to caution you about getting your hopes up too high." He dropped his voice slightly. "I don't think Viagra's going to work for you, Keith."

"Why not?" Keith asked, taken off guard. "It's supposed to be the cure-all, isn't it?"

"Well, that's what the media's been saying, but, in reality, there are many cases in which Viagra doesn't work, and I think your situation is one of them."

"Viagra works through the vascular system," Dr. Barrett explained. "It dilates the vessels to allow more blood flow to the penis. But your problem isn't just vascular. You have *physical* damage as well as vascular issues. And because of that, I think it's very likely you won't get any results from Viagra."

I was a bit disappointed, and Keith's expression registered the same.

"You're not alone in this regard, though," the physician hastened to add. "Over half the men I've written prescriptions for have told me it hasn't helped them either."

"Are you kidding me?" Keith was genuinely surprised. "*Half* the men you've treated can't use Viagra?"

"That's right. It's not something a lot of people realize. But then, you have to remember, most of the men I treat have serious medical problems. Many have had some kind of major surgery for their conditions. And this makes a big difference where impotence is concerned."

"But, I'm still going to give you the prescription," Dr. Barrett concluded more positively. "I could always be wrong, you know."

He wrote a hasty scrip and handed it to Keith.

Keith took the prescription and stood up. His face was now serious.

"I want you know how much I appreciate everything you've done for me," Keith said sincerely, gripping Dr. Barrett's hand. "For *everything* over the past four years—your persistence in urging me to get those biopsies and then persuading me to have that surgery. You saved my life…and I'm grateful."

Keith held his gaze while Dr. Barrett smiled and put his hand on Keith's shoulder, squeezing.

"Keith, it's been a pleasure to be a part of your recovery. I'm glad I've been able to help. Things have turned out well," he said with a satisfied grin. "And you deserve only the best."

Then the tall man turned and put his arms around me, squeezing me tight in a bear hug.

"You *both* deserve only the best!"

On our now-too-familiar ride home from the Clinic, Keith and I listened contentedly to classical music on NPR. I looked out the window, letting my mind drift with the music, and soon began to reminisce.

The gentle, sloping hillsides were green with newly emerging crops, yet I could remember three years ago, looking miserably out on this same scene and thinking that the winter farmsteads looked barren. I recalled how sad I was then.

And now look, I thought, they're budding with life again.

I turned to look at Keith sitting comfortably behind the steering wheel. He had lost weight since his surgery, and the shedding of those extra pounds made him look younger. No one would have guessed he had ever been sick or was anything less than totally healthy.

"Keith," I began slowly, "I know I've said this before, but I still can't get over how hard the last couple of years have been on our marriage. It was really scary. I just never thought we'd be so thrown by your impotence."

Keith glanced my way, and nodded in agreement.

"I know, babe. It's been rough all right."

I looked out the window again, and swallowed hard. Then I turned toward Keith once more.

"Keith, I'm really sorry for all the grief, I caused. I never wanted to hurt you," I said honestly.

Without answering, Keith slowed the car and pulled over to the side of the road. He switched off the engine, then turned to me and cupped my face in his soft warm hands, as he'd done so many times during our marriage.

He looked deep into my eyes.

"Gin," he said with tenderness, "we've both made mistakes and we've both done things we wish we hadn't, and we're *both* sorry. But we can't keep beating ourselves up over it."

He stroked the side of my face. "We've got to let it go and be grateful that we're happy again."

Keith gave me a playful kiss on the nose, then pulled back and landed another on my mouth.

"Who knows?" he joked, giving me that crooked boyish grin of his. "Maybe we'll be even happier with the Viagra!"

That night I put on my filmiest nightgown, lit candles and sprayed on perfume, while Keith shaved and combed his hair. We were looking forward to the evening, and doing our best to make everything as perfect as possible.

Despite the few minutes of skepticism at the Clinic, we were hopeful once again—hopeful that Viagra would work for us, that we could give up the shots and that we could have the luxury of making love anytime we wanted.

"I know it's silly, hon, but I actually feel a little nervous," I said as Keith came out of the bathroom, undoing his belt buckle. "Kind of like I'm going on a first date with you again or something."

"I know what you're saying," Keith laughed self-consciously. "I'm kind of nervous too—and I really don't know why."

We hugged each other. "How long has it been since you took it?" I whispered.

"Almost an hour ago. So anytime now should be fine," Keith smiled suggestively.

"Okay, I can't wait any longer. Let's go for it!"

I pulled Keith's hand and we rushed toward the bed.

"I can't believe this," Keith said disgustedly forty-five minutes later. "I'm going to take another pill."

Another pill.

Another forty-five minutes of foreplay.

But still, nothing doing.

"I'm so sorry it didn't work," I said, finally, laying back on my pillow.

"Yeah, me too," Keith replied, looking mournfully at his limp organ. "But it was worth the try."

The last song on the CD had finished playing long ago, and the room was quiet. But the smell of perfume and the flicker from the burning candles still permeated the air, filling it with the aura of possibility.

After a few minutes, Keith spoke.

"Gin," he murmured, "we can still rescue this night you know. If you want?"

"Oh yes," I said, turning toward Keith and giving his penis an anticipatory squeeze. "I'd love that. Let's do!"

Keith and I kissed—a slow, deep kiss. Then he went to give himself an injection.

When he returned, we whispered endearments and gently began touching each other.

We made love tenderly that night, with the love of over 30 years and the care of countless days to heighten our intimate knowledge of the other person's joy.

When we were finished, we slept peacefully.

Journal Entry, May 10, 1998

After two nights in a row, and four pills at a pop, we're convinced Viagra isn't going to work for Keith.

That's okay. It would have been nice to get away from the shots...but it's really no big deal <u>what</u> we use. The method has nothing to do, really, with "curing" impotence or being happy. That's something only <u>we</u> can accomplish. And that requires understanding, kindness and support for each other— not something that comes in a bottle.

So I guess we've got our <u>own</u> "miracle drug."

Laptop Notes, May 12, 1998

I would never have thought I could enjoy lovemaking like I do now.

I know I'm totally satisfying Gin, and she's fantastic for me. Its amazing how far we've come. We're really okay now.

I think of myself as recovered.

Looking Back
A New Definition of Intimacy

Gin, on intimacy...

Since dealing with the effects of impotence, I've changed my mind about the term "intimacy."

I used to think the real core of marital intimacy was the ability to confide in each other, which would in turn lead to a trusting relationship. I also thought that if one lost the ability to be sexual, it was all right—the marriage could still grow and thrive.

But I feel different now.

Today, the definition of marital intimacy, for me, *must* include physical sharing. I believe that Keith and I *have* to stay physically intimate with each other for our marital intimacy to survive—because when we don't, other facets of our marriage seem to suffer.

It must be understood, however, that I'm using the term "physical intimacy" in a broad sense. I can no longer think of physical intimacy as meaning only the "traditional" sexual experience. I also, however, cannot limit it to "just hugging"— not yet, anyway. Keith and I have talked about this a great deal, and we've decided that we define physical intimacy as "the intentional sharing of one's body for giving and receiving pleasure."

By "intentional" we mean that one is specific about engaging in the activity. By "pleasure" we mean "any physical act a couple agrees upon as being mutually satisfying."

While physical pleasure, for us, currently incorporates arousal and orgasm (usually), I do understand that there could come a time when circumstances dictate that we have to change our way of achieving physical pleasure. Perhaps only one of us might desire arousal. Perhaps we might have to go back to exclusively oral sex. Perhaps we'll someday arrive at a point where hugging *is* all we want to do.

But if and when such a time comes, I will try my best to live by my definition—making sure that, whatever we do, we've created a special time to totally concentrate on physically pleasing each other, and that whatever we do satisfies *each* of our needs.

These days the definition of intimacy, for us, is no longer as connected with *what* we do as much as with our *intentions*— to always keep some kind of sexual activity as a part of our lives.

Keith, on intimacy...

When I think of what the term "intimacy" means, I'm immediately reminded of the things I share with Gin that I wouldn't think of sharing with anyone else: my inner feelings, my insecurities, and, of course, my body. I suspect these are facets of a marital relationship that many people would consider the "intimate" ones.

It sounds simple, sharing these things with your partner, but it can get really complex. So many things can affect one's *willingness* to be intimate, and can cause a person to pull back.

When I look at the most difficult part of our recovery, I think one of the primary reasons we couldn't be intimate was because each of us was feeling a lack of safety.

I was hesitant to even *try* to make love with Gin because I was afraid I couldn't live up to her expectations. Gin says she was afraid to come on to me because she thought I was going to reject her (or be put in a position of seeming to have to "beg for it"). Basically, neither of us wanted to feel foolish.

Realizing this now, I understand that a major component of being intimate is feeling safe.

When Gin and I finally made our "contracts" with each other—the agreement to have consistent sex dates and the promise of not turning each other down—we had, without realizing it, created safe places. Only *then* were we able to begin the process of reestablishing our intimacy.

Recently, Gin asked me what advice I would give to people who have not had sexual relations in a long time. "It seems like it would be so difficult to even know how to *begin* being intimate again, if you haven't done anything in years," she pondered.

I agreed with her.

Here's my opinion. First, I think that a couple in this situation, or any couple really, who is dealing with sexual dysfunction, should consider getting professional counseling. The issue of sexual dysfunction is complex and, for me anyway, was an area where I really needed professional guidance.

Secondly, I would encourage couples in this situation to try to make safe places for themselves. I would encourage them to share their intimate thoughts and feelings on the subject with each other. Let your partner *hear* your fears, and *understand* your sense of feeling vulnerable.

When a safe place has been made, I would encourage couples to begin to share their bodies again, in *whatever way* they elect to do so.

Next to my recovery from cancer, I've found that reestablishing physical intimacy with Gin has been the greatest gift I've ever received. I love sharing my life with her again—body *and* soul.

EPILOGUE

Recovered, Happy and Sexual

Six years after Keith's surgery, and three years after what we consider to be our recovery, Keith and I continue to enjoy an exciting and energizing sexual relationship, very similar to what has been described in the last chapters of this book.

We still initiate lovemaking from a mental rather than physical drive, we continue to experiment and try new positions and devices, and we've consistently kept up with our sex dates— making love at least once every week (when we're together), for the past five years.

The consistency we've maintained in our lovemaking is amazing to us. Consistency has not been a common element in our marriage. We've each started at least six different diets, promised to keep to an exercise routine with no success, and still have projects left unfinished from years ago.

But in the area of our sex life, being consistent has seemed an easy task. We attend to our sex life because we really do believe it's as important to our marriage to be sexual as it is for our bodies to have food. Even when we don't "feel hungry," we maintain our physical "diet" to keep our marriage strong.

As with all couples, we've continued to face difficulties. Keith has had surgery for another cancer, I have had a complete hysterectomy. Keith's 85-year-old father is our primary responsibility now, and, at the same time, we're trying to make decisions about what to do with our own retirement.

But we've also never been happier.

We see each day as a gift. And impotence has taught us to treat each lovemaking experience as an added bonus.

We've learned to treasure the moment, but most importantly, we know we'll never stop making love again.

AFTERWARD

Fifteen Years Later

When MAKING LOVE AGAIN was published in 2002, Keith and I had overcome the social, physical and emotional consequences of Keith's impotence. We were making love again (enjoying intercourse) with the aid of penile injections and contentedly described our altered sexual life as our 'new normal.' All seemed well.

Life, however, does not stay static. In the fifteen years since the release of our book, much has changed. The penile injections which allowed Keith to achieve an erection stopped working. I dealt with the after effects of losing my libido after a hysterectomy. We have aged into our 70s.

Medicine and technology have also changed, especially in the area of sexual health. Improvements have been made in prostate cancer detection, allowing for cancers to be discovered earlier and treated with less invasive surgery. Penile implants (Keith now has one) require less extensive surgery and are 'more natural.' Women are now offered hormone therapy to ease the transition into menopause, and there are more lubrications available to help decrease discomfort during intercourse due to vaginal dryness that often accompanies aging. Breast cancer awareness and treatment have increased survival rates dramatically.

Life expectancy continues to increase, along with quality of health—which includes sexual health. And it is now accepted that most people can remain sexually active throughout their lifetime, and doing so can increase their overall well-being. Additionally, as a society we are become more accepting of diverse sexual preferences.

Yet speaking openly about sex and sexual dysfunction is still difficult for most people and couples. This is why our story remains relevant—because it deals with the emotional and relationship aspects of intimacy in a manner that encourages open dialogue and facilitates healing. It remains one of the few books written by a couple willing to share the good, bad, and even the ugly of dealing with sexual dysfunction. We have given the reader a front row seat to a critical phase in our marriage and how we got through the physical, psychological and emotional challenges of impotence—what we learned about 'making love' with and without intercourse, about the importance of touch, and most significantly the need for open, honest, explicit communication.

But I will repeat myself…life does not stay static. Keeping our intimate life healthy and active has been a continuous journey of evolution, adaptation, change, and discovery…especially as we have aged. So once again I'm writing with the same honesty and forthrightness I did in MAKING LOVE AGAIN.

I invite you to read the rest of the story on my website **virginialaken.com** as I post essays, resources, and conversations about intimacy and aging.

Virginia Laken
September 2017

About the Authors

Virginia Laken has retired from her communications consulting business but continues to publish. Her website is virginialaken.com. Keith has his own business, is a private pilot, and bee keeper. Married for 50 years, Keith and Virginia are proud parents of two grown children, five grandchildren, and a new great grandchild. They live in the rural Midwest.

To contact Virginia and Keith about your own experiences with sexual dysfunction, please visit hopeforcouples.com.

Sudafed® and Viagra® are registered trademarks of Pfizer, Inc.
Contac® is a registered trademark of GlaxoSmithKline.

ADDITIONAL NOTES

In writing one's own personal story, there is the constant question of what to include and what to leave out—with the goal being to keep the story interesting and engaging and still maintain accuracy. In that vein, I think we've done a good job of presenting our experience. But our experience is just that—only ours. And that made it impossible to present *all* the information on prostate cancer, impotence and related treatments that people might want to know.

Thus, I'd like to include a few comments here, at the end of our story, to give at least a hint of the many options that exist for dealing with either or both of these conditions.

We noted that, in the early '90s, when Keith was investigating treatment options for prostate cancer, the primary treatments available were surgery, external-beam therapy (radiation), and watchful waiting. Today, those options have been expanded, and a partial listing could also include interstitial brachytherapy (the implantation of radioactive seeds), cryoblation (freezing the cancer cells within the prostate), and proton-beam therapy (another form of radiation). There are also various forms of hormone therapy that could be considered and/or a combination of the above. (For a more thorough investigation of prostate cancer treatment options, as well as possible side effects, please consult the Resources section of this book.)

In the treatment of erectile dysfunction, it must again be noted that there were options available at the time that Keith and I did not consider. These methods would include vacuum erection devices (VEDs), penile implants, penile suppositories containing medication similar to the injections and a tourniquet-type ring (often referred to as a "cock ring").

And then there was Viagra—the first oral medication for the treatment of impatience, which Keith and I did try, but with no success.

The search for a "cure" for impotence continues. Shortly after the printing of this book, there should be two *new* oral medications on the market. Cialis, which is being developed by Lilly ICOS LLC, is being touted as having more "staying power" than Viagra—meaning that a man should be able to get an erection *any* time within 24 hours of taking the drug. Bayer's new drug, generically called vardenafil at present, is also coming to market shortly, and may cause fewer side effects than Viagra. Additionally, hormone therapy may help some men to achieve erection, either used on its own or in combination with one or more of the other treatments.

Some of the better-known medical treatments for impotence are generally recommended or prescribed by a urologist or general practitioner. But I feel I must also note some of the other, adjunct professionals and practitioners who play a crucial role in successfully treating erectile dysfunction. These specialists include endocrinologists, psychologists, psychiatrists, mental health therapists and marital health professionals—all of whom have experience in dealing with sexual dysfunction. These people generally advocate treatment that includes the man *and* his partner, and address the significant emotional aspect of erectile dysfunction. When this aspect is not addressed, it often keeps the purely "medical" approach from becoming a lasting and satisfying cure.

ACKNOWLEDGEMENTS

Prior to writing this book, I had no idea how mentally and emotionally draining it could be to tell a story. Nor did I appreciate the importance of support and encouragement from others. Now that I *do* recognize these things, I'd like to publicly thank the people who have helped me accomplish this task.

First, I must acknowledge the support given to me from my children. Beth and Steven did more than just encourage—they were active, involved participants in my efforts. Beth spent days cloistered in a motel room with me, sorting through the bits and pieces of my thoughts, and patiently listening to *hours* of revisions, ever willing to offer insight. Steven has always been ready to lift my spirits, and has been an excellent medical resource, as well as a proud promoter of the book. Faithfully reminding me of the importance of this project, our children have been mindful that this book could ease the heartache of others.

Next, I want to recognize three highly talented women, who offered their skills, advice and, most importantly, their friendship. Rita Faro helped me with the initial organization of this book. Her enthusiasm was incredible and has *never* waned. Rita's energy and positive nature pulled me out of the dumps more than once. Judy Wilkinson helped to fine-tune the original manuscript, adding life, interest and depth. Her ability to get to the heart of issues allowed me to find gems of insight. Maria Bishop, my editor from Ant Hill Press, suggested the wonderful addition of the "Looking Back" sections. Her quick mind immediately saw voids in the copy, and her persistence in finding "just the right words" has made this book even more focused and readable. To each of these individuals, I give my heartfelt thanks.

Other women who deserve my thanks for their support and encouragement are the members of the International Women's Writers Guild—expecially the founder, Hannelore Hahn, and Susan Tiberghien, Eunice Scarf and Alison Strickland.

My appreciation also goes to Ant Hill Press, and its publisher, George Trim. George was willing, not only to take a chance on publishing a book about a highly sensitive subject, but also to work with a first-time author. He has been remarkably patient teacher and a wise manager.

I must also express gratitude to friends and family, who have been so understanding throughout this process. You respected my need to draw back for a while and focus my attention on writing, and, at the same time, you were supportive and encouraging. I've missed our time together, and I'm looking forward to reconnecting again!

Finally, I must recognize my collaborator and dear husband, Keith. Without Keith's strength, this book would never have happened. He has shown remarkable courage in being able to put the needs of others above his own, discussing a very personal subject with a respectfulness I admire. Keith, you have always been my most steadfast supporter and strongest ally, and I am a better person because of you.

—Virginia Laken

BIBLIOGRAPHY

Alterowitz, Ralph and Barbara. *The Lovin' Ain't Over: The Couple's Guide To Better Sex After Prostate Disease.* Westbury, New York: Health Education Literary Publishing, 1999.

Barrett, David M., M.D., ed. *Mayo Clinic on Prostate Health.* Rochester, Minnesota: The Mayo Clinic, 2000. Distributed by Kensington Publishing Corp., New York, 2000.

Cutler, Winnifred B., Ph.D. *Love Cycles, The Science Of Intimacy.* New York: Villard Books, a division of Random House, Inc., 1991.

Dorso, Michael A., M.D. *Seeds of Hope.* Battle Creek, Michigan: Acorn Publishing, A Project Division of Development Initiatives, 2000.

Godat, Joseph L., M.D. *Putting Impotence To Bed: What Every Man & Woman Need To Know.* Arlington, Texas: The Summit Publishing Group, 1999.

Gray, John, Ph.D. *Mars And Venus In The Bedroom: A Guide To Lasting Romance and Passion.* New York: HarperCollins, 1995.

Hooper, Anne. *Anne Hooper's Kama Sutra: Classic Lovemaking Techniques Reinterpreted For Today's Lovers.* New York: Dorling Kindersley Inc., 1994.

Kantoff, Philip W., ed., Wishnow, Kenneth I. M.D., ed., and Loughlin, Kevin R. M.D. *Prostate Cancer: A Multidisciplinary Guide.* Malden, Massachusetts: Blackwell Science Inc., 1997.

Keesling, Barbara, Ph.D. *Sexual Pleasure: Reaching New Heights of Sexual Arousal and Intimacy.* Alameda, California: Hunter House Inc., 1993.

Moore, Thomas. *The Soul of Sex: Cultivating Life as an Act of Love.* New York: HarperPerennial, a division of HarperCollins, 1998.

Morganstern, Steven, M.D. and Abrahams, Allen E., Ph.D. *The Prostate Sourcebook: Everything You Need to Know.* Los Angeles: Lowell House, 1998.

Ridley, Matt. *The Red Queen: Sex And The Evolution Of Human Nature.* New York: Penguin Books USA, 1995.

Stanway, Andrew M.D., *The Lovers' Guide: The Art of Better Lovemaking.* New York: St. Martin's Press, 1994.

Stoff, Jesse A., M.D. and Clouatre, Dallas, Ph.D. *The Prostate Miracle: New Natural Therapies That Can Save Your Life!* New York: Kensington Publishing Corporation, 2000.

Walsh, Patrick C., M.D. and Farrar Worthington, Janet. *The Prostate: A Guide For Men And The Women Who Love Them.* Baltimore: The Johns Hopkins University Press, 1995.

Resources

Mayo Clinic
www.mayoclinic.org
Male and female sexual dysfunction treatment specialists.

University of Minnesota Center for Sexual Health
www.sexualhealth.umn.edu
Advancing the sexual health of Minnesota, the nation, and the world through preeminence in research, education, clinical service, and advocacy.

Center for Sexual Function – part of the Lahey Clinic in Boston, Massachusetts
www.impotence-center.com
This excellent website explains the purpose of the Center for Sexual Function, which also includes a "Frequently Asked Questions" link regarding sexual functioning for both men and women.

Sexuality Information and Education Council of the United States
www.siecus.org
This site contains an excellent bibliography on sexuality issues for older adults, with a listing of valuable resources for facing the physical and emotional changes and challenges of middle and later life.

Queendom.com
www.queendom.com
Personality and IQ tests, quizzes and personality tests.

The New Prostate Cancer Infolink Social Network
prostatecancerinfolink.net

The "New" Prostate Cancer InfoLink has been developed to become a primary source of accurate, current, and topical information about prostate cancer for patients and their families.

US TOO! News You Can Use
www.ustoo.com
This informative website cites current articles on prostate cancer and the effects of both the disease and its treatments, including erectile dysfunction.

First To Know Bulletin
www.ivanhoe.com/firsttoknow
This is a good medical source containing hundreds of current medical news reports. Searches can be customized by interest, and therefore can include searches for information on erectile dysfunction.

Medscape Urology
www.medscape.com/urology
Medscape will send weekly mailings to subscribers, with the latest information on prostate cancer, erectile dysfunction or any related urologic condition including drugs, therapies, studies and research associated with these conditions.

American Foundation For Urologic Disease
www.afud.org
This is an extensive site created exclusively for the treatment of urological diseases, offering a wide range of valuable information on erectile dysfunction. The site also provides links to a host of other informative and useful sites on the subject.

The Circle
www.prostatepointers.org/circle/
This interactive support group is for wives/partners, families and friends of men with prostate cancer, as well as for the men themselves. Nancy Peress monitors this site, and every Friday sends out a compiled list of Internet resources for members.

These resources are most useful, and the shared information from "real" people can be a comfort as well as a source of inspiration. A subgroup deals specifically with the effects, issues and challenges of impotence.

Us Too

www.ustoo.org

This interactive support group is for wives/partners, families and friends of men with prostate cancer, as well as for the men themselves.

Salon.com

www.salon.com

This website features articles, products, news reports and reviews on a broad base of sexual topics and subjects. The diversity of this site may be helpful in broadening the imagination and stretching one's perspective.

ORGANIZATIONS:

American Cancer Society

National Cancer Institute Cancer Information Services

Sexual Function Health Council

American Association of Sex Educators, Counselors and Therapists

www.aaset.org

American Diabetes Association, National Center

www.diabetes.org

American Heart Association National Center

www.heart.org

American Menopause Foundation Inc.
www.menopause.org

American Society on Aging
www.asaging.org

National Kidney and Urologic Diseases Information Clearing House
healthinaging.org/resourcenational

INDEX

Incontinence, see also Catheter,
Prostate Cancer Surgery,
28-30, 37-39, 134
Injections, see also Impotence,
Manliness, Sex, Sex Life,
Scarring, 5, 67-77, 79, 82-83,
89-97, 105, 113-115, 118,
124-125, 127, 129-130,
132-133, 135-136, 143, 149,
153, 156, 160-161, 171
Intercourse, see also
Experimentation, Impotence
and sex, Sex, Lovemaking,
34, 55, 58, 59, 75, 90, 129,
147, 149, 150, 153, 164
Intimacy, see also
Experimentation, Impotence,
Lovemaking, Marriage,
Relationship, Sex, 32, 34, 42,
46, 51, 146, 152-153, 161,
164-166
Johns Hopkins, 6, 18, 21, 155
Journal Entries, xiv, 5-6, 16,
21, 23, 25, 28-29, 32-33, 39,
43, 56, 60, 69-70, 77, 89-91,
95, 99-100, 103-104,
108-109, 115-116, 122-123,
128, 131, 135, 144-145, 148,
150, 161-162
Kama Sutra, see also
Experimentation, 57
Libido, see also Arousal, Desire,
Mind-Body Connection, Sex,
Sex Drive, 96, 98, 117,
120-124, 135, 138-139

Love Potion, see also Injections,
77, 92
Lovemaking, see also
Experimentation, Impotence,
Marriage, Relationship, Sex,
2, 15, 25-26, 32-34, 39, 42,
46, 51, 55-57, 59-60, 62, 70,
75, 91-92, 99, 101, 104-105,
120, 127, 128-130, 133-136,
138, 143, 145, 147, 149-150,
153, 156, 161-162, 165, 167
Male Sexual Dysfunction, see
Sexual Dysfunction
Manliness, see also
Depression, Eunuch,
Performance Anxiety, Self
Deprecation, Self Image, 3-4,
33, 54, 89, 92, 94-95, 121,
123, 145
Marriage, see also Impotence,
Intimacy, Counseling,
Relationship, Sex, Quality of
Life, 4, 6, 11-12, 31, 33-34,
37, 51, 58, 62, 67, 84,
106-108, 112-113, 116, 119,
127, 129, 145-146, 150, 155,
159, 164, 167
Massage, see also Arousal,
Experimentation, 58, 93
Masturbation, see also
Experimentation, Oral Sex,
Sex, Vibrator, 33, 39, 129
Mayo Clinic, 3, 7, 9, 16, 19-20,
39, 71, 73-76, 80, 84, 118,
131, 157, 159-160

Prostate Cancer, see also Practitioner-Patient Interaction, xiii, xv, 1-8, 10, 12, 14-17, 19-23, 26-27, 39-40, 48, 52-53, 61, 64, 84, 102, 112, 115, 117, 132, 134, 142, 146, 150, 152, 157, 166, 168, 171

and diagnosis, see also Biopsy, PSA, 1, 13-16, 18-19, 82, 102, 145, 149

and impotence, see impotence

and recovery, see also Recovery, Remission, 27, 39, 117, 132, 142-143, 145, 166

and treatment, see also Counseling, Radiation, Surgery, Treatment, Watchful Waiting, 3, 10, 17, 21-22, 48-49, 152, 171

Prostate Cancer Surgery, see also Nerve-Sparing Technique, Prostate Cancer and treatment, 1, 3, 6, 10, 12-13, 16-22, 25-29, 32, 34, 38-39, 51, 53, 58-59, 61, 64, 68-69, 82, 87, 95, 97, 120, 130, 134-135, 138, 158-159, 167-168, 171

Prostate Cancer Support Group, 18-20, 61-62

Prostate Specific Antigens, see PSA

Prostatectomy, see also Prostate Cancer Surgery, 19, 28, 68, 139

PSA, see also Prostate Cancer and diagnosis, 3, 8, 22, 39-40, 77, 131-132, 157

Psychiatry, see also Rome, M.D., Rosen, Raymond PhD., 115, 117

Psychology, see also Williams, Donald PhD., xii, 58, 119, 121, 124, 172

Quality of Life, see also Counseling, Depression, Journal Entries, Marriage, Recovery, Relationship, Sex, Sex Life, Well-Being, 132

Radiation, see also Healing, Impotence, Prostate Cancer and recovery, Quality of Life, 18, 27-28, 33, 37-39, 55, 65, 86, 100, 117, 119, 124, 130, 132, 136, 138, 142-143, 145, 158, 165-167

Relationship, see also Counseling, Impotence and relationship, Intimacy, Marriage, Prostate Cancer and Relationship, Sex and relationship, Sex Life, Quality of Life, xiv, xv, 11, 33-35, 52, 64-67, 86, 92-101, 105-106, 112-124, 127, 143-150, 152, 156-157, 159, 164-168

Remission, see also Prostate Cancer and recovery, 22, 142

Rome M.D., see also Counseling, 115, 117, 119

Rosen, Raymond PhD., 124

Stricture, see also Prostate
Cancer Surgery, 68, 70-71
Sudafed, see also Decongestant,
Priapism, 80, 84, 91, 169
Surgery, see Prostate Cancer
Surgery
Therapy, see also Counseling,
Radiation, 16
Treatment, see also Impotence
and treatment, Prostate
Cancer and treatment, 3, 10,
17, 21-22, 48-49, 71, 125,
139, 152, 156, 171-172
Urology, see also Barrett, David,
M.D., xiii, 7-8, 76, 80, 83,
172
Williams, Donald PhD., see
also Counseling, Psychology,
118-125, 127, 130-131, 133,
138, 143, 145-146

Vascular Damage, 158
Viagra, see also Impotence and
treatment, 155-158, 160, 169,
171-172
Vibrator, see also
Experimentation, 32, 156
Watchful Waiting, see also
Prostate Cancer and
treatment, 3, 8, 171
Well-Being, see also
Counseling, Depression,
Quality of Life, Relationship,
7, 34, 65

FURTHER READING

For more by Virginia and Keith Laken, please visit:

hopeforcouples.com

virginialaken.com

Made in the USA
Coppell, TX
26 May 2020